PRP FOR SHOULDER PAIN

A PATIENT'S GUIDE TO PLATELET-RICH PLASMA THERAPY & RECOVERY

FIRST EDITION / MMXXVI

JOSHUA B ROTHENBERG DO
ROBERT ENGELEN DO
DAVID ESPINOZA MD
JOSE RAMIREZ-DEL TORO MD

PRP FOR SHOULDER PAIN

A PATIENT'S GUIDE TO PLATELET-RICH PLASMA THERAPY & RECOVERY

FIRST EDITION / MMXXVI

BLACK BEAR
SOLUTIONS 1

ISBN: 979-8-9963475-0-6 (eBook)
979-8-9963475-1-3 (paperback)

Published in the United States by

Black Bear Solutions 1, LLC
Fort Lauderdale, Florida

Editing, Proofreading, and Interior/Layout Design by
ThoroughProof Services

ACKNOWLEDGMENTS

We would like to express our sincere gratitude to everyone who contributed to the creation of this book.

Special thanks go to our illustrator, Vishal Ashok Gokuwale, whose creativity, talent, and dedication helped bring these pages to life. Their artistic vision added depth, character, and meaning to the work in ways that words alone could not.

We are also deeply grateful to our family and friends for their unwavering support, encouragement, and patience throughout this journey. Their belief in us provided the inspiration and strength needed to bring this project to completion.

Finally, we wish to honor the memory of our late mentor, Gerard Malanga. His guidance, wisdom, and generosity left a lasting impression on our lives and work. Though he is no longer with us, his influence continues to inspire us, and this book stands as a testament to the lessons he shared and the example he set.

To all who helped, supported, and inspired us along the way, we offer our heartfelt thanks.

ABOUT THE AUTHORS

Joshua Rothenberg, DO, FAAPMR, CAQSM, is a double board-certified physician in Physical Medicine & Rehabilitation and Sports Medicine and the founder of Rothenberg Orthopedics, Regenerative and Sports Medicine in Boca Raton, Florida. He completed fellowship training at the University of Pittsburgh Medical Center (UPMC) and has received national recognition for his work in musculoskeletal medicine, orthobiologics, and ultrasound-guided procedures. Dr. Rothenberg is an international lecturer, published researcher, and author of *A Beginner's Guide to Musculoskeletal Ultrasound*, with a passion for advancing evidence-based, non-surgical orthopedic care.

Robert Engelen, DO, FAAPMR, CAQSM, is a board-certified Physical Medicine and Rehabilitation physician with fellowship training in Sports Medicine from the University of Pittsburgh Medical Center. A former U.S. Navy lieutenant and battalion medical officer for 1st Battalion, 6th Marines, he deployed to Afghanistan and was awarded the Navy and Marine Corps Commendation Medal and the Combat Action Ribbon. Dr. Engelen specializes in sports medicine, orthobiologics, minimally invasive procedures, and performance optimization. He has served as a team physician for the Utah Royals and as Assistant Team Physician for Real Salt Lake. He lives in Salt Lake City, Utah, with his wife and three children and enjoys skiing, mountain biking, jiu-jitsu, and coaching youth sports.

David Espinoza, MD, is a board-certified physician in Sports and Family Medicine, currently in private practice at TSAOG Orthopedics & Spine in San Antonio, Texas. He completed fellowship training at the University of Pittsburgh Medical Center (UPMC), where he subsequently served as assistant professor and team physician for Robert Morris University. At TSAOG, he established the non-surgical sports medicine program, served as team physician for the San Antonio Missions Double-A baseball team, and is a clinical professor at the University of the Incarnate Word (UIW) School of Medicine. His clinical focus includes ultrasound-guided procedures and orthobiologic therapies to provide non-surgical treatment of orthopedic conditions, emphasizing care delivered with integrity, presence, and a goal of restoration and vitality.

Jose Ramirez-Del Toro, MD, is board-certified in Physical Medicine and Rehabilitation and subspecialty board-certified in Sports Medicine. He completed his Sports Medicine Fellowship at New Jersey Sports Medicine Associates (now the New Jersey Regenerative Institute) under the mentorship of the late Dr. Gerard Malanga. Dr. Ramirez-Del Toro previously served as Sports Medicine Fellowship Director at the University of Pittsburgh and currently practices in private practice. He lectures nationally and has authored numerous book chapters on musculoskeletal ultrasound, interventional procedures, and platelet-rich plasma therapies.

Prathap Jayaram, MD, is a Professor of Physical Medicine and Rehabilitation and Orthopedics at the University of Michigan, where he serves as Associate Chair and Director of Nonoperative Sports Medicine. He specializes in sports medicine, musculoskeletal care, and regenerative orthobiologics, with research focused on osteoarthritis, tendon disorders, and translational musculoskeletal science. Dr. Jayaram is nationally recognized for his clinical, research, and leadership contributions to advancing nonoperative orthopedic care.

Peter A. Everts, PhD, is an internationally recognized scientist, educator, and thought leader in regenerative medicine, orthobiology, and outcomes optimization. He holds academic appointments as Adjunct Professor at The University of Queensland Medical School (Australia) and Professor at UniMAX Medical School (Brazil), where he also serves as lecturer and instructor in regenerative medicine. Dr. Everts is a Fellow of the Royal Society of Medicine (UK), a founding board member of the International Regenerative Medicine Experts Society (IARMES), and Scientific Lead of the European Network Organization Regenerative Medicine (ENORM). As Founder and CEO of Everts Scientific, he focuses on advancing evidence-based regenerative therapies and translating scientific innovation into improved clinical outcomes worldwide.

Stephen Schaaf, MD, RMSK, is an Assistant Professor of Physical Medicine and Rehabilitation at Vanderbilt University Medical Center, where he practices sports medicine with a clinical focus on musculoskeletal ultrasound. He completed residency training in Physical Medicine and Rehabilitation and fellowship training in Sports Medicine at the University of Pittsburgh Medical Center, with clinical and academic interests in musculoskeletal disorders, image-guided interventions, and the application of ultrasound in sports and rehabilitation medicine.

Megan Ferderber, MD, MPH, is a sports medicine physician with extensive experience in both medical education and clinical practice. A graduate of Penn State College of

Medicine in Hershey, PA, she completed her Family Medicine residency at UPMC St. Margaret, where she served as co-chief, and subsequently remained at UPMC for a Sports Medicine fellowship. She is board-certified in Family Medicine, Sports Medicine, and Lifestyle Medicine, holds a Master of Public Health degree, and is certified in musculoskeletal ultrasound (RMSK). She currently practices as a sports medicine physician at the Lehigh Valley Orthopedic Institute (LVHN) in Northeast Pennsylvania.

Christopher Urbanek, DO, is a sports medicine physician specializing in interventional orthobiologics and regenerative medicine. A graduate of the Philadelphia College of Osteopathic Medicine (PCOM), he completed his Family Medicine residency and Sports Medicine fellowship at UPMC St. Margaret. He further advanced his training through a second fellowship in Interventional Orthobiologics of the Spine and Extremities at the Centeno-Schultz Clinic and is certified in Regenerative Medicine and Interventional Pain Management through the American Board of Interventional Pain Physicians (ABIPP). Dr. Urbanek is dedicated to advancing patient education and promoting the evidence-based use of orthobiologic therapies, including platelet-rich plasma (PRP) and cell-based treatments.

Glenn M. Flanagan, MD, is a physician specializing in orthobiologics and regenerative medicine and serves as the Founder and Medical Director of Naples Regenerative Institute. His clinical and academic work focuses on platelet-rich plasma (PRP), bone marrow concentrate, and advanced image-guided musculoskeletal interventions. Dr. Flanagan has contributed to peer-reviewed publications and textbook chapters and is dedicated to advancing evidence-based regenerative medicine through innovation, precision, and outcomes research.

Gayan Poovendran, MD, CAQSM, is a dual board-certified family medicine and sports medicine physician and Co-Founder of PRO Institute, a regenerative sports medicine practice with locations in Davie and Miami Shores, Florida. He specializes in non-surgical orthopedic care, including platelet-rich plasma (PRP), autologous cell-based therapies, and peptide optimization for joint, tendon, and ligament injuries. Dr. Poovendran is an educator and speaker known for helping golfers and athletes worldwide remain active, optimize performance, and avoid surgery whenever possible.

Joe Fiorelli, PT, DPT, is the National Director at BARWIS Physical Therapy and a Board-Certified Sports Clinical Specialist—a distinction held by less than 2% of physical therapists nationwide. He specializes in orthopedics, musculoskeletal care, and sports rehabilitation, focusing on individuals ranging from professional athletes to recreational movers. Dr. Fiorelli's clinical focus extends beyond traditional symptom management, aiming to surpass a patient's pre-injury baseline and achieve optimal, long-term physical health.

Kelly Fiorelli, PT, DPT, CSCS, is a Director of Physical Therapy at Barwis Physical Therapy. As a physical therapist and Certified Strength and Conditioning Specialist, she has played a key role in the growth and development of Barwis Physical Therapy as a nationally recognized leader in rehabilitation and performance. Kelly specializes in helping individuals recover from injury, improve movement, and build lasting strength through evidence-based exercise and training.

Austin Sturdivant, MD, is completing his Physical Medicine and Rehabilitation residency at Vanderbilt University Medical Center, where he currently serves as chief resident. He earned his medical degree from the University of Tennessee Health Science Center (UTHSC) College of

Medicine and completed his undergraduate studies at the University of Memphis.

Michael Diaz Greenberg, MD, is completing his Physical Medicine and Rehabilitation residency at Vanderbilt University Medical Center. He earned his medical degree from Vanderbilt University and completed his undergraduate studies at the University of Central Florida. Following residency, Dr. Greenberg plans to pursue a fellowship in sports medicine.

Sarah Allen is a medical student at the University of Ottawa with a focused interest in rehabilitation and recovery following injury and illness. She has contributed to several research projects in these areas and has presented her work at academic conferences. She plans to pursue a career in Physical Medicine and Rehabilitation. This represents her first contribution to a book-length academic publication.

TABLE OF CONTENTS

PREFACE

Author: Joshua Rothenberg, DO

As a clinician with extensive experience in regenerative medicine, I have observed a significant surge of interest in innovative therapies designed to enhance the body's intrinsic healing capabilities. Platelet-Rich Plasma (PRP) therapy stands out as a particularly promising treatment within this evolving field, especially for musculoskeletal conditions. This interest is further fueled by the field's rapid advancements and the increasing number of scientific studies and clinical applications being explored across various medical specialties. The autologous nature of PRP, coupled with its favorable safety profile, relatively low cost, and minimally invasive application, contributes to its growing acceptance among both patients and clinicians. Despite its growing popularity, there are numerous common concerns and misconceptions surrounding PRP therapy among patients and the general public. These often stem from a lack of clear understanding regarding its precise mechanisms of action, perceived effectiveness, and safety. Patients may harbor fears about potential side effects or question its efficacy due to inconsistent terminology and varied preparation methods that contribute to heterogeneous clinical outcomes. This book aims to address these widespread concerns by offering comprehensive, research-backed guidance to empower patients with an informed understanding of PRP therapy for shoulder conditions. By synthesizing findings from high-quality clinical studies and systematic reviews, the book provides evidence that PRP therapy can lead to significant improvements in pain relief and functional outcomes for common shoulder ailments, such as rotator cuff injuries and frozen shoulder, amongst others. Comparative studies have also demonstrated that PRP can offer promising longer-term benefits in reducing pain and disability associated with conditions like osteoarthritis when compared to traditional treatments. This approach ensures that the guidance provided is grounded in current, peer-reviewed research, enabling patients to make well-informed decisions about PRP as a non-surgical, regenerative option for managing shoulder pain.

Understanding Shoulder Pain and PRP's Role

Shoulder pain is a frequently reported musculoskeletal complaint, impacting a substantial segment of the adult population at some point in their lives. The shoulder's complex anatomy, which allows for a wide range of motion while maintaining stability, also makes it vulnerable to various injuries and conditions that cause pain and functional limitations. Common causes of shoulder pain include rotator cuff injuries, arthritis, bursitis, labral tears, and frozen shoulder. Rotator cuff injuries are a primary cause of shoulder pain and dysfunction, encompassing conditions from tendinitis and tendinopathy to partial and full-thickness tears, with the supraspinatus muscle being most frequently affected. Arthritis, including osteoarthritis and inflammatory types, contributes to chronic pain and stiffness due to degenerative changes in joint cartilage and inflammation. Bursitis, such as subacromial-subdeltoid bursitis, results from inflammation of the bursa, causing localized pain that worsens with shoulder movement. Labral tears involve injuries to the cartilage lining the shoulder socket, leading to pain and mechanical symptoms. Frozen shoulder, also known as adhesive capsulitis, is characterized by progressive pain and severe restriction of shoulder motion due to capsular fibrosis and inflammation.

Despite the prevalence of these conditions, traditional treatments for shoulder pain, such as corticosteroid injections, nonsteroidal anti-inflammatory drugs (NSAIDs), and surgery, often provide only temporary relief or do not adequately promote long-term healing. Corticosteroid injections, while effective for short-term pain reduction, typically offer benefits for less than 12 weeks, and repeated use carries risks such as tendon weakening and potential adverse effects on rotator cuff healing. NSAIDs, although they alleviate pain and inflammation, are associated with systemic side effects and primarily mask symptoms without addressing tissue regeneration. Surgical interventions, while necessary in some severe cases, are invasive, require lengthy recovery periods, and do not always guarantee full restoration of tissue health or prevent disease progression.

Platelet-Rich Plasma (PRP) therapy offers a novel approach that addresses the limitations of traditional treatments by fitting into modern orthopedic practice as a non-surgical, regenerative option. PRP harnesses the body's natural healing capabilities by delivering a concentrated dose of platelets, growth factors, and cytokines to the injured area. These biological components stimulate cellular processes crucial for tissue repair and regeneration, including cell proliferation, collagen synthesis, angiogenesis, and inflammation modulation, thereby promoting intrinsic healing rather than merely alleviating symptoms. This approach allows for enhanced functional recovery, reduced recovery times, and potentially decreases the need for more invasive procedures. As an autologous therapy, derived from the patient's own blood, PRP also minimizes risks of hypersensitivity or infection. Its ability to stimulate biological healing makes PRP a promising alternative for individuals seeking a more restorative treatment for various musculoskeletal conditions.

Who Can Benefit from PRP?

Platelet-Rich Plasma (PRP) therapy may be beneficial for several patient populations, offering a non-surgical avenue to promote a healing environment. Active individuals with overuse injuries, such as tendinopathies and other musculoskeletal conditions common in athletes and physically active people, are often ideal candidates. PRP has demonstrated promise in promoting tissue repair and accelerating recovery in these cases, facilitating a faster return to activities and potentially mitigating complications.

Furthermore, patients who have failed conservative treatments, including physical therapy, nonsteroidal anti-inflammatory drugs (NSAIDs), or steroid injections, may find PRP therapy to be an effective second-line option. PRP is considered a promising intervention for chronic tendinopathies and joint conditions where first-line therapies have not yielded sufficient relief or regenerative benefits.

Athletes at all levels, from recreational to professional, frequently choose PRP therapy to expedite the healing of tendon, ligament, muscle, and cartilage injuries. This therapeutic modality aims to reduce downtime and improve functional recovery, making it a valuable tool in sports medicine.

However, PRP therapy may not be suitable for all individuals. It is generally not ideal for patients with severe joint degeneration where extensive structural damage necessitates surgical intervention, as PRP is more effective in promoting healing in mild to moderate cases. Individuals with bleeding disorders or those currently on anticoagulant therapy are typically not ideal candidates due to the increased risk of complications related to platelet dysfunction or impaired clotting. Other contraindications for PRP use include active infections, tumors, metastatic disease, thrombocytopenia, anemia, pregnancy, and lactation. Therefore, a thorough screening for these conditions is essential to ensure the safety and optimize the efficacy of PRP treatments.

Picture of an injection of PRP into the shoulder

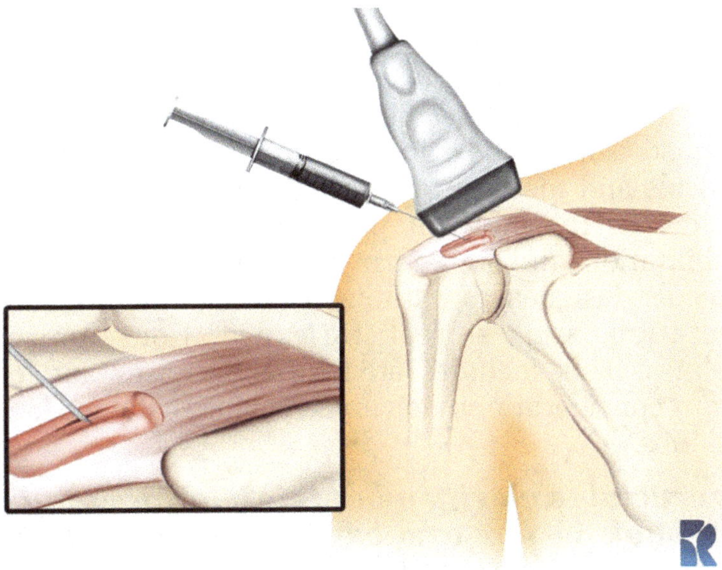

Setting Expectations for This Book

This book is carefully crafted to serve as a comprehensive resource primarily for patients who are considering or currently undergoing Platelet-Rich Plasma (PRP) therapy for shoulder conditions. It is also designed to be a valuable tool for healthcare providers, offering insights that can enhance their understanding and discussions with patients. The book is organized into clear, structured sections that simplify complex medical information, making it accessible to a broad audience. Each section integrates current, research-backed knowledge with practical, actionable advice, empowering readers to make informed decisions about their treatment options.

The main topics covered include the science behind PRP, explaining its biological composition of growth factors and cytokines, and how these elements facilitate tissue repair and regeneration. It details the mechanisms by which PRP influences healing processes and modulates inflammation within damaged tissues. The book also thoroughly explains the PRP treatment process, from patient selection and indications to the specifics of how PRP is prepared and administered, emphasizing the importance of standardized protocols and medical professionalism to ensure safety and efficacy. Furthermore, it provides extensive guidance on rehabilitation and long-term recovery, outlining post-PRP protocols designed to optimize healing, enhance functional restoration, and set realistic expectations for recovery timelines. This includes advice on exercises and physical therapy considerations vital for achieving sustained long-term outcomes.

It is crucial to clarify what this book does not cover. This book is not a substitute for direct medical advice. Patients should always consult their healthcare providers for personalized diagnoses and treatment recommendations tailored to their specific individual conditions and medical history. While PRP therapy has an expanding range of applications across various medical fields, this book focuses exclusively on its use in shoulder pathology and does not delve into PRP applications beyond shoulder conditions. For information on broader or

alternative uses of PRP therapy, it is advisable to consult other specialized resources or medical professionals.

CHAPTER 1

Understanding PRP Therapy

Authors: Joshua Rothenberg, Glenn Flanagan & Jose Ramirez-Del Toro

What is Platelet-Rich Plasma (PRP)?

Platelet-Rich Plasma (PRP) is an autologous blood product characterized by a concentration of platelets significantly higher than the baseline levels found in whole blood. Its therapeutic application stems from the fact that these concentrated platelets are a rich source of various growth factors and bioactive proteins. These factors play a pivotal role in supporting the natural wound healing and tissue repair cascades, encompassing inflammation, proliferation, and remodeling phases. PRP therapies are increasingly recognized as an adjunctive treatment in regenerative medicine for conditions such as musculoskeletal and spinal disorders, osteoarthritis, and chronic wounds. The appeal of PRP lies in its autologous origin, which largely disregards concerns of disease transmission or immunogenic reactions.

Distinguishing Blood Components

To fully comprehend PRP, it is essential to differentiate it from other blood components. Whole blood is the complete, unprocessed blood drawn from a patient, consisting of cellular elements like red blood cells, white blood cells, and platelets, all suspended within a liquid matrix called plasma. Plasma, also known as blood plasma, is the light-yellowish or straw-colored liquid component that serves as the base for whole blood and transports cells, proteins, and other substances throughout the body. Platelets, or thrombocytes, are anucleated cell fragments produced from megakaryocytes in the bone marrow, primarily recognized for their critical role in primary hemostasis (blood clotting) and thrombosis. Beyond clotting, platelets are increasingly identified as significant modulators of inflammation and tissue regeneration due to their ability to store and release a diverse array of biologically active components, including growth factors, cytokines, and chemokines. Platelet-Rich Plasma (PRP), therefore, is a specific fraction of plasma where the concentration of these vital platelets is significantly elevated above physiological baseline values through a processing technique, typically centrifugation, to enhance its regenerative potential for targeted therapeutic applications.

Derivation of Platelet-Rich Plasma: The Centrifugation Process

The derivation of PRP involves a precise process that begins with the extraction of blood from the patient, which is then collected into tubes usually containing anticoagulants like acid citrate dextrose (ACD-A) or sodium citrate to prevent clotting during preparation. The collected blood undergoes a centrifugation process, which separates the blood into its constituent layers based on their differing densities. The heaviest components, red blood cells, settle at the bottom, followed by a middle layer known as the buffy coat, which is rich in leukocytes (white blood cells) and platelets, with the lightest component, plasma, at the top.

Different centrifugation protocols are employed, with the most common being single-spin and double-spin methods. In a single-spin protocol, blood is centrifuged once at a specific speed and duration to separate components, resulting in PRP with varying platelet and leukocyte concentrations depending on the parameters. The double-spin method, often preferred for its ability to achieve higher platelet concentrations and better control over cellular composition, involves two distinct centrifugation steps. The first, a "soft" spin, separates red blood cells from the plasma, while keeping platelets and leukocytes suspended in the plasma. This platelet- and leukocyte-rich plasma is then transferred to a new tube and subjected to a second, "hard" spin to pellet the platelets at the bottom. The supernatant, platelet-poor plasma (PPP), is then removed, leaving a highly concentrated platelet-rich plasma for extraction. The final step involves PRP extraction, where the concentrated PRP is carefully collected for therapeutic injection into the target tissue. Variations in centrifugation speed, duration, and the type of anticoagulant significantly influence the quantity and quality of the obtained PRP, affecting factors such as platelet count, cell recovery rates, and the composition of other components like leukocytes.

PRP Formulations: Leukocyte-Rich vs. Leukocyte-Poor and Concentration Variations

Platelet-Rich Plasma formulations vary considerably, particularly regarding their leukocyte (white blood cell) content, leading to classifications such as Leukocyte-Rich PRP (LR-PRP) and Leukocyte-Poor PRP (LP-PRP). LR-PRP contains a higher concentration of leukocytes along with platelets, which can induce an initial pro-inflammatory response due to the presence of inflammatory cytokines like IL-1β and TNF-α from activated leukocytes. This inflammation may be beneficial in some contexts to stimulate healing, but can also lead to increased post-injection pain or swelling. Conversely, LP-PRP is processed to minimize leukocyte content, aiming to reduce inflammatory mediators, and is often preferred where inflammation needs to be less pronounced. Studies show that LP-PRP may significantly reduce re-tear rates and improve clinical results in certain repairs compared to LR-PRP. However, LR-PRP can express significantly more anti-inflammatory mediators like IL-1Ra, IL-4, and IL-8, suggesting potential benefits for long-term chronic low-grade inflammation, although it may also contain higher concentrations of MMP-9, which can be chondrotoxic.

The platelet concentration in PRP also varies widely, typically ranging from 1 to 10 times the baseline concentration, but may get higher in the 15 to 20 times range of whole blood, depending on the preparation method. Higher platelet concentrations are generally associated with a greater release of growth factors essential for tissue repair, such as Platelet-Derived Growth Factor (PDGF), Transforming Growth Factor Beta (TGF-β), Vascular Endothelial Growth Factor (VEGF), Epidermal Growth Factor (EGF), and Insulin-like Growth Factor-1 (IGF-1). However, the optimal platelet concentration is still under investigation, and clinical outcomes do not always directly correlate with the highest platelet count, indicating the complexity of PRP's biological effects. Commercial PRP preparation systems contribute to this variability, offering different centrifugation protocols, speeds, and times, and some systems include filters for leukodepletion. The lack of consensus and standardization in PRP preparation methods across various devices makes it challenging to compare research findings and optimize clinical protocols.

How PRP Works: The Role of Platelets in Tissue Healing

Platelets are pivotal regulators of wound healing and tissue regeneration, extending their role beyond primary hemostasis. Upon injury and activation, platelets undergo a transformative process, releasing over 300 biologically active components from their granules. These include a myriad of growth factors, cytokines, and chemokines, which sequentially promote neovascularization, restore damaged connective tissue, and facilitate the proliferation and differentiation of mesenchymal stem cells into tissue-specific cell types.

Key growth factors found in platelets, such as Platelet-Derived Growth Factor (PDGF), Transforming Growth Factor Beta (TGF-β), Vascular Endothelial Growth Factor (VEGF), Epidermal Growth Factor (EGF), and Insulin-like Growth Factor-1 (IGF-1), are crucial for cell proliferation, migration, and angiogenesis. PDGF, for instance, stimulates cell proliferation and is important for recruiting cells to the repair site. TGF-β plays an important role in the inflammatory phase and promotes tissue fibrosis and collagen production, which are vital for extracellular matrix remodeling. VEGF is essential for angiogenesis, the formation of new blood vessels, which improves blood supply and nutrient delivery to damaged tissues. EGF stimulates epithelial cell growth and differentiation, critical for wound closure. IGF-1 supports cellular growth, metabolism, and aging, and is involved in reducing inflammation and promoting cartilage repair.

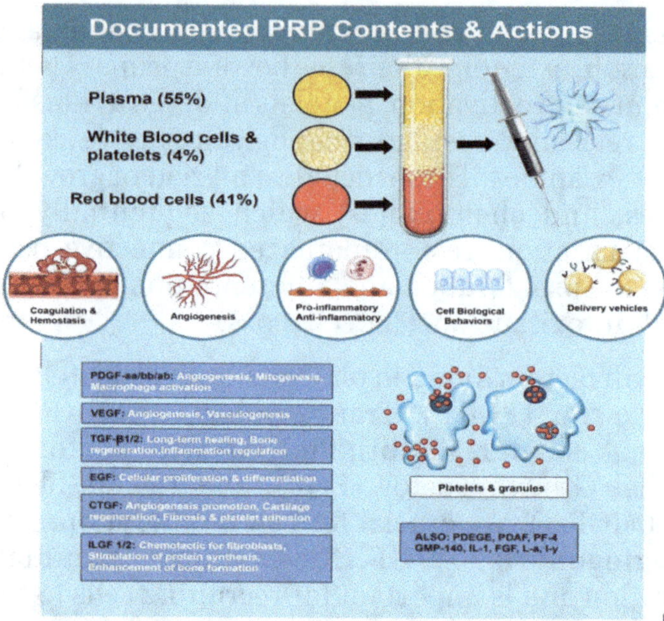

Figure 1.1 Components and Biological Activities of Platelet-Rich Plasma (PRP)

PRP profoundly influences inflammation, tissue regeneration, and pain modulation. It modulates inflammation by regulating macrophage polarization, promoting a shift from pro-inflammatory M1 to anti-inflammatory M2 phenotypes, and reducing levels of pro-inflammatory cytokines such as TNF-α and IL-1β. This contributes to both tissue repair and an analgesic effect. In terms of tissue regeneration, PRP enhances angiogenesis, as seen by increased vessel formation, and boosts collagen production, particularly collagen type I, which is crucial for the structural integrity and strength of healing tissues. Moreover, PRP stimulates stem cell recruitment and proliferation, attracting reparative cells to the injury site and influencing their differentiation into tissue-specific cell types, thereby accelerating tissue repair.

Biological Timeline After PRP Injection

The biological events following a PRP injection unfold in a predictable timeline, initiating a cascade of healing processes. Within the first 24 hours, platelets within the injected PRP are activated, releasing a concentrated burst of growth factors and cytokines. This immediate release, including PDGF, TGF-β, VEGF, EGF, and IGF-1, initiates the inflammatory phase of healing. During this period, PRP also helps modulate the initial inflammatory response, attracting immune cells like macrophages and stimulating early fibroblast activity, which prepares the wound environment for subsequent repair.

Within 7 days post-injection, the proliferative phase becomes dominant. The sustained presence of growth factors continues to drive angiogenesis, leading to the formation of new blood vessels that supply vital oxygen and nutrients to the healing tissue. Fibroblasts actively proliferate and increase collagen synthesis, particularly the initial formation of Type III collagen, which forms a foundational extracellular matrix scaffold. Concurrently, PRP-derived factors enhance stem cell recruitment and their subsequent proliferation and differentiation, contributing directly to tissue regeneration.

Beyond 7 days, the remodeling phase begins and can extend for weeks to months, depending on the tissue and severity of injury. In this phase, the initially laid collagen matrix is reorganized and matured, transitioning from weaker Type III collagen to stronger Type I collagen, thereby improving the mechanical strength and function of the repaired tissue. PRP's early influence helps guide this remodeling process, often leading to better tissue quality and reduced scar formation compared to natural healing alone. This sustained reparative process contributes to long-term pain relief and functional improvement by facilitating structural tissue restoration.

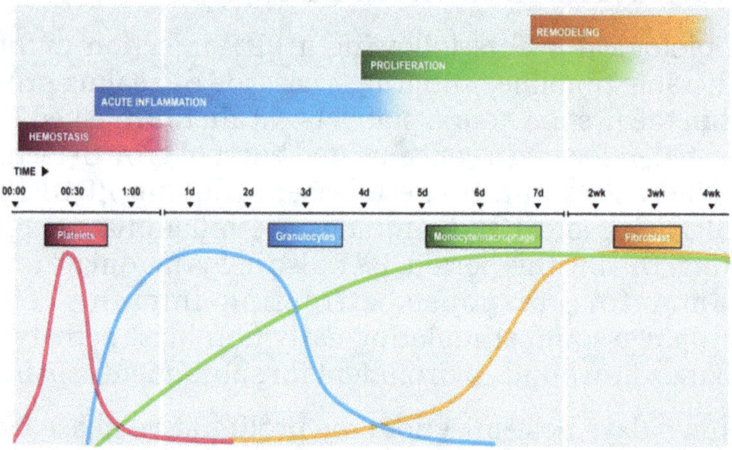

Figure 1.2 Temporal Phases of Tissue Healing and Cellular Activity Following Injury

PRP vs. Other Treatments (Steroid Injections, Surgery, Physical Therapy)

Comparison with Cortisone: Quick Relief vs. Long-term Tissue Effects

When considering treatments for musculoskeletal conditions, Platelet-Rich Plasma (PRP) therapy and cortisone (corticosteroid) injections present distinct profiles regarding pain relief and long-term tissue effects. Corticosteroid injections are widely recognized for their ability to provide rapid, short-term pain relief, often within days to weeks, due to their potent anti-inflammatory properties. This immediate symptomatic relief makes them a common choice for acute pain and inflammation. However, the benefits of steroid injections are typically transient, with relief often diminishing over weeks to a few months. Furthermore, concerns exist regarding their long-term impact on tissue health, as repeated steroid use can potentially accelerate cartilage degeneration, impair soft tissue healing, and lead to adverse effects like tendon weakening or tissue atrophy.

In contrast, PRP focuses on a regenerative approach, harnessing the body's natural healing mechanisms. While PRP may not provide the immediate pain relief seen with corticosteroids, its effects typically lead to superior and more sustained improvements in pain and function over longer periods, often becoming more noticeable after several months. PRP achieves this by delivering concentrated growth factors that modulate inflammation and actively promote tissue repair, including enhanced collagen synthesis and angiogenesis. Studies comparing PRP and corticosteroids for conditions like knee osteoarthritis, lateral epicondylitis, and plantar fasciitis indicate that while steroids may offer quicker initial relief, PRP often yields better long-term outcomes in pain control and functional recovery. For example, in carpal tunnel syndrome, PRP injections demonstrate superior and safer long-term efficacy compared to steroids. In sacroiliac joint pain, PRP is considered safer, despite steroids providing more immediate relief.

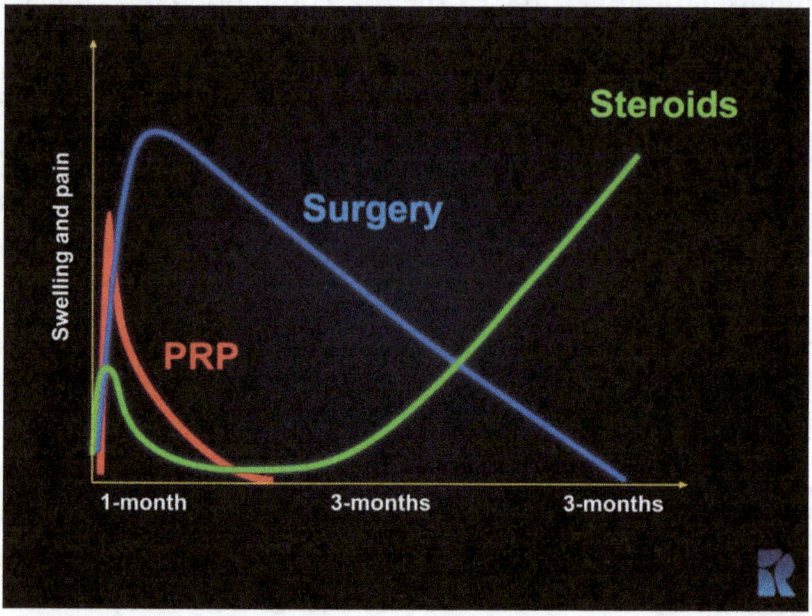

Figure 1.3 Conceptual Symptom Response Over Time Following PRP, Corticosteroid Injection, and Surgery

PRP Compared to Surgery: Delaying or Preventing Surgical Needs

PRP therapy is emerging as a valuable non-surgical intervention that can delay or, in certain scenarios, prevent the need for more invasive surgical procedures. Its regenerative capabilities offer an alternative, particularly in early to moderate stages of degenerative diseases and musculoskeletal injuries. For instance, in knee osteoarthritis, PRP injections have been shown to significantly delay the need for knee arthroplasty, offering a valid treatment to postpone or potentially avoid surgery. Similarly, for post-traumatic ankle osteoarthritis, PRP has demonstrated effectiveness in improving symptoms and deferring the necessity for invasive surgical interventions.

For various tendinopathies like tennis elbow, PRP injections have proven to be a safe and effective tool that can potentially eliminate the need for surgical intervention. Even in complex fields like orthodontics, PRP application has shown promise in accelerating treatment outcomes. While surgery remains a definitive solution for severe or refractory cases, PRP's ability to promote natural tissue repair, modulate inflammation, and enhance healing makes it a compelling option for patients seeking fewer invasive treatments that can effectively manage their conditions and potentially delay or even preclude surgical intervention.

Physical Therapy's Role as a Complement, Not a Competitor

Physical therapy plays a crucial complementary role to PRP therapy, working synergistically to optimize patient outcomes rather than acting as a competing treatment. While PRP therapy provides the biological stimulus for tissue regeneration by delivering concentrated growth factors, physical therapy focuses on the biomechanical and functional aspects of recovery. Through targeted exercises, manual therapy, and rehabilitation protocols, physical therapy helps restore joint mobility, muscle strength, and overall function, which directly supports and enhances the regenerative processes initiated by PRP.

This combined approach is often more effective than either therapy alone. For instance, in patients with knee osteoarthritis, PRP combined with physical therapy can lead to significant improvements in pain and functional scores. Physical therapy aids in improving range of motion and tissue conditioning, facilitating proper healing and integration of the newly regenerated tissues. It can also help to prevent re-injury by improving strength, stability, and movement patterns. Essentially, PRP creates a biological environment to promote healing, and physical therapy then leverages this improved environment to rebuild function and durability, ensuring comprehensive and sustained recovery.

Long-term Safety Profile of PRP vs. Steroids and NSAIDs

Platelet-Rich Plasma (PRP) therapy generally boasts a favorable long-term safety profile, largely due to its autologous nature, meaning it is derived from the patient's own blood. This minimizes the risk of allergic reactions, disease transmission, or severe adverse immune responses. Common adverse effects associated with PRP injections are typically mild and localized, such as transient pain, redness, or swelling at the injection site. Research consistently indicates a low risk of morbidity associated with intra-articular PRP injections in large joints like the knee, hip, and shoulder.

In comparison, corticosteroid injections, while providing rapid symptomatic relief, are associated with a range of potential short-term and long-term adverse effects. These include possible tissue atrophy, weakening of tendons, and risks associated with repeated use, such as cartilage damage. Systemic side effects, such as elevated blood sugar levels, can also occur, particularly for patients with pre-existing conditions like diabetes. The anti-inflammatory action of corticosteroids does not promote tissue regeneration and may, in fact, hinder the natural healing process over time.

Non-Steroidal Anti-Inflammatory Drugs (NSAIDs), used for pain and inflammation management, carry systemic risks, especially with chronic use. These can include gastrointestinal issues (e.g., ulcers), cardiovascular complications, and renal impairment. While topical or oral NSAIDs can provide pain relief, they do not contribute to tissue regeneration. In contrast, PRP avoids these systemic risks by acting locally and stimulating the body's intrinsic healing and regenerative processes. This makes PRP an attractive alternative for long-term management of chronic conditions, as it aims to repair the underlying pathology rather than just suppressing symptoms, all while maintaining a low-risk profile.

Comparison Chart

PRP therapy demonstrates a unique profile of regenerative potential combined with a low-risk and minimally invasive approach. Unlike steroids, which may provide rapid but short-lived relief without healing properties, PRP actively promotes a tissue healing environment, potentially delaying or avoiding the need for surgery. While surgery remains a definitive option for severe conditions, it carries higher risks and a longer recovery. Physical therapy complements these treatments by aiding functional recovery and should be considered part of a comprehensive care plan.

Table 1.1 PRP vs. Other Treatments: Comparison Chart

Treatment	Mechanism	Relief Onset	Tissue Healing	Duration of Effect	Safety	Role in Surgery	Complement with PT
PRP Therapy	Promotes healing via growth factors and cytokines	Gradual (weeks to months)	Promotes regeneration (collagen, angiogenesis)	Long-lasting pain and function improvement	Excellent; autologous and low risk	Can delay or avoid surgery	Works synergistically with PT for better outcomes
Steroid Injections	Suppresses inflammation and immune response	Fast (days)	May impair tissue over time	Short-lived (weeks to months)	Risk of tissue atrophy, tendon weakening, systemic effects	Palliative, not preventative	Temporary aid for PT
Surgery	Physically repairs or removes damaged tissue	Post-op recovery dependent	Corrects structure but does not regenerate tissue	Often permanent, but with long rehab	Higher risk (infection, anesthesia, complications)	Definitive for severe/refractory cases	Requires PT post-operatively
Physical Therapy	Restores biomechanics through movement	Gradual and progressive	Improves load tolerance and recovery support	Sustained with adherence	Very safe with minimal risk	Helps prevent or recover from surgery	Primary therapy or combined with PRP

Key Takeaways and Recap

Platelet-Rich Plasma (PRP) is a natural, autologous regenerative therapy derived from the patient's own blood. It concentrates platelets along with growth factors and cytokines essential for tissue repair and regeneration. Biologically, PRP works by releasing key growth factors such as PDGF, TGF-β, VEGF, and EGF, which initiate and promote inflammation modulation, enhance cellular proliferation, stimulate angiogenesis, and recruit stem cells to the injured tissue. This process facilitates collagen production and accelerates a healing environment. Unlike steroid injections that provide rapid but often temporary pain relief with potential negative effects on tissue integrity, PRP offers long-term regenerative benefits by promoting natural tissue healing without the adverse effects associated with steroids and NSAIDs. In comparison to surgery, PRP may serve as a less invasive option to delay or prevent surgical intervention by enhancing the body's intrinsic healing mechanisms. Physical therapy complements PRP therapy by supporting functional recovery, but PRP targets regenerative processes directly at the cellular and molecular levels. PRP has a superior safety profile with minimal risks and side effects given its autologous nature, making it an attractive alternative or adjunct to traditional treatments.

As we conclude Chapter 1 and prepare to delve deeper into the specific conditions that PRP therapy can help address, remember that understanding the foundational science and comparison with other treatments is crucial. This knowledge empowers you to make informed decisions tailored to your unique health needs. Embrace this journey towards enhanced wellness and let us continue together to discover how PRP can be a transformative part of your health care plan.

Bibliography

Aboalola, D., Ramadan, M., & Baadhaim, M. (2024). Public awareness and understanding of stem cell treatments available in Saudi Arabia and their trust in hospitals and research centers involved in stem cell research. *Frontiers in Public Health*, *12*, Article 1364809. https://doi.org/10.3389/fpubh.2024.1364809

Aborukbah, A. F., Ashoor, M. M., Elbashir, H. A., Namri, S. T., Hamdi, E. A., Khayat, Z. M., Sharahili, R. M., Alharbi, N., Fallatah, A. S., & Balqurun, H. M. (2024). Comparative imaging modalities for diagnosing rotator cuff injuries. *International Journal of Community Medicine and Public Health*, *11*(4), 1735–1742. https://doi.org/10.18203/2394-6040.ijcmph20240999

Acute shoulder pain—Common causes and their management. (2018). *National Health and Medical Research Council Guidelines*, *41*(2), 112–118.

Akan, O., Mete, B., Yılmaz, H., & Tosun, A. (2019). Efficacy of ultrasound guided platelet-rich plasma in the repair of partial and full-thickness supraspinatus tears. *Journal of Back and Musculoskeletal Rehabilitation*, *32*(6), 871–878. https://doi.org/10.3233/BMR-181245

Annaniemi, J., Pere, J., & Giordano, S. (2021). Platelet-rich plasma versus corticosteroid injections in rotator cuff related shoulder pain: A comparative study with up to 18 months of follow-up. *Journal of Orthopaedics*, *24*, 152–158. https://doi.org/10.5397/cise.2021.00486

Anwar, J., Ali, U., Akbar, W., Shaheen, F., Ahmad, I., & Ullah, K. (2017). Platelet-rich plasma (PRP) therapy for osteoarthritis of the knee joint recent updates and future perspectives. *Journal of Postgraduate Medical Institute*, *31*(4), 345–351.

Arita, S., & Tobita, M. (2024). Adverse events related to platelet-rich plasma therapy and future issues to be resolved. *Regenerative Therapy*, *26*, 375–381. https://doi.org/10.1016/j.reth.2024.05.011

Banday, M., & Muzaffar, J. (2018). The effect of platelet-rich plasma injection on lateral epicondylitis following failed conservative management. *International Journal of Orthopaedics Sciences*, *4*(2), 193–197. https://doi.org/10.22271/ortho.2018.v4.i2d.33

Barman, A., Mishra, A., Maiti, R., & Sahoo, J. (2021). Can platelet-rich plasma injections provide better pain relief and functional outcomes in persons with common shoulder diseases: A meta-analysis of randomized controlled trials. *Journal of Clinical Orthopaedics and Trauma*, *23*, Article 101625. https://doi.org/10.1016/j.jcot.2021.101625

Barham, R. (2019). *Guides: ASTU 3030: Computers in the visual arts: Books*. University of North Texas Libraries. https://library.unt.edu

Belcinski, D. (2020). Psychological treatment of medical patients struggling with harmful substance use. *Journal of the Medical Library Association*, *108*(4), 675–676. https://doi.org/10.5195/jmla.2020.1068

Brinkman, J. C., McQuivey, K. S., & Hassebrock, J. D. (2023). Public interest in shoulder platelet-rich plasma injections is increasing: A 10-year Google Trends analysis. *JSES International*, *7*(4), 633–638. https://doi.org/10.1016/j.jseint.2023.02.006

Buchheit, T., Huh, Y., Maixner, W., Cheng, J., & Ji, R. (2020). Neuroimmune modulation of pain and regenerative pain medicine. *Journal of Clinical Investigation*, *130*(11), 5635–5648. https://doi.org/10.1172/JCI140065

Cauwenberghe, E. V. (2017). *Technology and business trends in regenerative medicine*. Frost & Sullivan.

Charliyan, G. (2023). PRP therapy for the treatment of sacral fracture and coccydynia: A case report. *Pain Medicine Case Reports, 7*(4), 145–149.

Chaudhary, S. K., & Meena, S. (2024). Revolutionizing orthopedics: The role of regenerative medicine in healing and repair. *International Journal for Multidisciplinary Research, 6*(1), 1–9. https://doi.org/10.36948/ijfmr.2024.v06i01.12185

Cole, B. J., Cotter, E. J., Wang, K. C., & Davey, A. (2017). Patient understanding, expectations, and satisfaction regarding rotator cuff injuries and surgical management. *Arthroscopy: The Journal of Arthroscopic & Related Surgery, 33*(8), 1603–1611. https://doi.org/10.1016/j.arthro.2017.03.024

Cook, T., & Lewis, J. (2019). Rotator cuff–related shoulder pain: To inject or not to inject? *Journal of Orthopaedic & Sports Physical Therapy, 49*(5), 289–293. https://doi.org/10.2519/jospt.2019.0607

Cooper-Moss, N., Hooper, H., Choong, K., & Chauhan, U. (2021). Medical professionalism: Navigating modern challenges. *InnovAiT, 14*(12), 743–749. https://doi.org/10.1177/17557380211052669

Dalili, D., Bansal, T., Khandwalla, N., Shah, Z., George, M., Bankes, M., & Isaac, A. (2017). Traumatic overuse injuries in athletes: An observational nonrandomised prospective study with multimodality imaging and follow up. *British Journal of Sports Medicine, 51*(4), 312–313. https://doi.org/10.1136/bjsports-2016-097372.63

de Castro, J. C. (2022). Regenerative medicine procedures under ultrasound guidance. In J. C. de Castro (Ed.), *Ultrasound-guided musculoskeletal procedures* (pp. 235–252). Springer. https://doi.org/10.1007/978-3-

030-98256-0_14

De Pieri, A., Rochev, Y., & Zeugolis, D. I. (2021). Scaffold-free cell-based tissue engineering therapies: Advances, shortfalls and forecast. *npj Regenerative Medicine, 6*(1), Article 18. https://doi.org/10.1038/s41536-021-00133-3

Demeco, A., de Sire, A., Salerno, A., Marotta, N., Palermi, S., Frizziero, A., & Costantino, C. (2024). Dry needling in overhead athletes with myofascial shoulder pain: A systematic review. *Sports, 12*(6), Article 156. https://doi.org/10.3390/sports12060156

ElgharibAbouelmaaty, M., Nassar, W. A. M., Hussein, A., & Allam, A. (2021). The effect of ultrasound guided platelet rich plasma (PRP) injection in the non-surgical treatment of partial supraspinatus tendon tear. *The Egyptian Journal of Hospital Medicine, 85*(1), 3290–3296. https://doi.org/10.21608/ejhm.2021.196582

Elshenawy, E. A., Nassar, I., Elkhouly, R., & Dabees, N. (2021). MRI and ultrasonography in the evaluation of causes of shoulder pain. *Tanta Medical Journal, 49*(1), 22–29. https://doi.org/10.4103/tmj.tmj_32_20

Emer, J. (2019). Platelet-rich plasma (PRP): Current applications in dermatology. *Skin Therapy Letter, 24*(5), 1–6.

Everts, P., Onishi, K., Jayaram, P., & Lana, J. F. (2020). Platelet-rich plasma: New performance understandings and therapeutic considerations in 2020. *International Journal of Molecular Sciences, 21*(20), Article 7794. https://doi.org/10.3390/ijms21207794

Everts, P. A., van Erp, A., DeSimone, A., & Cohen, D. S. (2021). Platelet-rich plasma in orthopedic surgical medicine. *Platelets, 32*(2), 163–174.

https://doi.org/10.1080/09537104.2020.1869717

Eymard, F., Louati, K., Noel, É., & Abouqal, R. (2025). Indications and contraindications to platelet-rich plasma injections in musculoskeletal diseases in case of infectious, oncological and haematological comorbidities: A systematic review. *Joint Bone Spine*, *92*(1), Article 105782. https://doi.org/10.1016/j.jbspin.2024.105782

Faltesek, D. (2019). How to use this book. In R. Molina-Pérez & A. Larramendi (Eds.), *Dinosaur facts and figures: The theropods and other dinosauriformes* (pp. 6–7). Princeton University Press. https://doi.org/10.1515/9780691194691-002

Fang, J., Wang, X., Jiang, W., Zhu, Y., & Hu, Y. (2020). Platelet-rich plasma therapy in the treatment of diseases associated with orthopedic injuries. *Tissue Engineering Part B: Reviews*, *26*(6), 571–585. https://doi.org/10.1089/ten.teb.2019.0292

Filardo, G., Previtali, D., Napoli, F., & Candrian, C. (2021). PRP injections for the treatment of knee osteoarthritis: A meta-analysis of randomized controlled trials. *Cartilage*, *13*(1_suppl), 364S–375S. https://doi.org/10.1177/1947603520931170

Fukui, S., Rokutanda, R., Kawaai, S., & Suda, M. (2023). Current evidence and practical knowledge for ultrasound-guided procedures in rheumatology: Joint aspiration, injection, and other applications. *Best Practice & Research Clinical Rheumatology*, *37*(3), Article 101852. https://doi.org/10.1016/j.berh.2023.101852

Gallicchio, V. S. (2023). Stem cell therapy for rotator cuff injuries. *Journal of Regenerative Medicine & Biology Research*, *4*(1), 1–12.

Gentile, P., & Garcovich, S. (2020). Systematic review—The

potential implications of different platelet-rich plasma (PRP) concentrations in regenerative medicine for tissue repair. *International Journal of Molecular Sciences*, *21*(16), Article 5702. https://doi.org/10.3390/ijms21165702

Goddard, N. V., & Waterhouse, N. (2020). Regenerative medicine, stem cell therapies, and platelet-rich plasma: Where is the evidence? *Aesthetic Surgery Journal*, *40*(4), 460–462. https://doi.org/10.1093/asj/sjz351

Gonçalves, N., Frantz, N., & de Oliveira, R. (2020). Platelet-rich plasma (PRP) therapy: An approach in reproductive medicine based on successful animal models. *Animal Reproduction*, *17*(2), Article e20180093. https://doi.org/10.21451/1984-3143-AR2018-093

Gorodilova, A. V., Kharisova, C. B., Osinnikova, M. N., Kitaeva, K., Filin, I. Y., Mayasin, Y. P., Solovyeva, V., & Rizvanov, A. (2024). The well-forgotten old: Platelet-rich plasma in modern anti-aging therapy. *Cells*, *13*(11), Article 942. https://doi.org/10.3390/cells13211755

Gupta, S., Paliczak, A., & Delgado, D. (2021). Evidence-based indications of platelet-rich plasma therapy. *Expert Review of Hematology*, *14*(1), 97–108. https://doi.org/10.1080/17474086.2021.1860002

Heidari, N., Slevin, M., Zeinolabediny, Y., Meloni, D. J., Olgiati, S., Wilson, A., Noorani, A., & Azamfirei, L. (2022). Comparison of the effect of MFAT and MFAT + PRP on treatment of hip osteoarthritis: An observational, intention-to-treat study at one year. *Journal of Clinical Medicine*, *11*(4), Article 1056. https://doi.org/10.3390/jcm11041056

Hilton, L. (2018). The latest research on PRP. *Dermatology Times*, *39*(8), 34–36.

Hoogland, M. A. (2019). How medical students discover and

use medical information tools. *Medical Reference Services Quarterly*, *38*(3), 235–248. https://doi.org/10.1080/02763869.2019.1623407

Jaseem, M., Alungal, S., Dhiyaneswaran, & Shamsudeen, J. (2020). Effectiveness of autologous PRP therapy in chronic nonhealing ulcer: A 2-year retrospective descriptive study. *Journal of Family Medicine and Primary Care*, *9*(9), 4799–4803. https://doi.org/10.4103/jfmpc.jfmpc_611_20

Jayaram, P., Yeh, P. C., & Cianca, J. (2019). Platelet-rich plasma protocols can potentiate vascular emboli: Contraindications to platelet-rich plasma. *Journal of International Society of Physical and Rehabilitation Medicine*, *2*(2), 67–71. https://doi.org/10.4103/jisprm.jisprm_12_19

Kossev, A., & Sokolov, T. (2018). Platelet-rich plasma (PRP) in orthopedics and traumatology. *Journal of IMAB - Annual Proceeding (Scientific Papers)*, *24*(4), 2268–2272. https://doi.org/10.5272/jimab.2018244.2268

Kourosh, A. S., Mangual, K. P. S., Farah, R. S., & Rao, M. (2024). Platelet-rich plasma: Advances and controversies in hair restoration and skin rejuvenation. *Dermatologic Surgery*, *50*(5), 415–422. https://doi.org/10.1097/DSS.0000000000004132

Kumar, A., Singh, M. S., & Rani, B. (2020). Effect of platelet rich plasma (PRP) injection in shoulder having partial rotator cuff tears. *International Journal of Orthopaedics Sciences*, *6*(2), 524–527. https://doi.org/10.22271/ortho.2020.v6.i2i.2116

Lambert, M. (2023). How to make friends and influence people? Lancaster Medical Book Club and professional leadership in the early NHS. *Morecambe Bay Medical Journal*, *9*(4), 112–116.

https://doi.org/10.48037/mbmj.v9i4.1354

Le, A. D. K., Enweze, L., DeBaun, M. R., & Dragoo, J. L. (2018). Current clinical recommendations for use of platelet-rich plasma. *Current Reviews in Musculoskeletal Medicine*, *11*(4), 624–634. https://doi.org/10.1007/s12178-018-9527-7

Lee, K. (2023). Medical professionalism version 2.0. *Korean Journal of Medical Ethics*, *26*(1), 45–62. https://doi.org/10.35301/ksme.2023.26.1.45

Lee, Y. (2021). Evaluation of shoulder pain in outpatient clinic. *Korean Journal of Family Practice*, *11*(4), 243–251. https://doi.org/10.21215/kjfp.2021.11.4.243

Lyles, E., Stegura, C., Broughton, L., Snyder, A., & Schlesinger, T. (2024). Basic science and principles of stem cells, platelet-rich plasma, and exosomes. *Dermatological Reviews*, *5*(2), 87–99. https://doi.org/10.1002/der2.217

Magalon, J., Brandin, T., Francois, P., & Degioanni, C. (2021). Technical and biological review of authorized medical devices for platelets-rich plasma preparation in the field of regenerative medicine. *Platelets*, *32*(7), 882–891. https://doi.org/10.1080/09537104.2020.1832653

Magruder, M., & Rodeo, S. A. (2021). Is antiplatelet therapy contraindicated after platelet-rich plasma treatment? A narrative review. *The Orthopaedic Journal of Sports Medicine*, *9*(5). https://doi.org/10.1177/23259671211010510

Makarevich, P. I., & Tkachuk, V. A. (2024). Fundamental and practical perspectives in regenerative medicine. *International Journal of Molecular Sciences*, *25*(4), Article 2004. https://doi.org/10.3390/ijms25042004

Masilamani, N., & Ganapathy, D. (2020). Awareness about regenerative therapy with of platelet-rich plasma (PRP) among dental students. *International Journal of*

Research in Pharmaceutical Sciences, 11(SPL3), 1194–1198. https://doi.org/10.26452/ijrps.v11iSPL3.3364McNamee, M. J., Coveney, C. M., Faulkner, A., & Gabe, J. (2018). Ethics, evidence based sports medicine, and the use of platelet rich plasma in the English Premier League. *Health Care Analysis, 26*(3), 241–261. https://doi.org/10.1007/s10728-017-0345-7

McNamee, M., Coveney, C. M., Faulkner, A., & Gabe, J. (2018). Ethics, evidence based sports medicine, and the use of platelet rich plasma in the English premier league. *Health Care Analysis, 26*(4), 344–361. https://doi.org/10.1007/s10728-017-0345-7

Medical professionalism. (2025). In *Oxford textbook of medical education* (2nd ed.). Oxford University Press. https://doi.org/10.1093/med/9780198871637.003.0005

Mehta, S., Bishnoi, A., & Dogra, S. (2022). Regenerative medicine in aesthetics. *CosmoDerma, 2*, Article 105. https://doi.org/10.25259/CSDM_46_2022

Mishra, S., Kaur, D., & Dhanda, M. (2022). Ultrasound-tailored treatment of subacromial shoulder pain: Exploring the role of platelet-rich plasma versus steroids. *Global Journal of Transfusion Medicine, 7*(2), 154–160.

Mlachkova, A., Dosseva-Panova, V., & Popova, C. (2021). Application of PRP (platelet-rich plasma) in surgical periodontal therapy: Overview. *Biotechnology & Biotechnological Equipment, 35*(1), 1234–1244.

Muzatarovna, M. M. (2024). PRP therapy significantly reduces urinary incontinence severity and improves quality of life. *European Journal of Medical Genetics and Clinical Biology, 1*(2), 74–79.

Nadeau-Vallée, M., Ellassraoui, S., & Brulotte, V. (2025). Platelet-rich plasma injections as a second-line treatment in patients with tendinopathy-related chronic pain and failure of conservative treatment: A systematic review and meta-analysis. *Pain Medicine*, *26*(3), 412–425. https://doi.org/10.1093/pm/pnaf022

Niazy, A. H. M., Ali, A. H., & Mahmoud, M. (2020). Role of ultrasound guided injection of platelet-rich plasma (PRP) in rotator cuff tendinopathy. *QJM: An International Journal of Medicine*, *113*(Suppl 1), hcaa104-006.

Olifirenko, O., Hertsen, H. I., Movchan, O., Serhiienko, R., Protsyk, A., & Ostapchuk, R. (2021). Method to obtain PRP and L-PRP for the use in routine medical practice of orthopedic traumatologist. *Trauma*, *22*(4), 38–44.

Parvez, Z., Akter, S., & Shobnom, A. T. (2021). Usefulness of PRP therapy in androgenic alopecia. *European Journal of Medical and Health Sciences*, *3*(4), 45–49.

Patil, P., Jadhav, M., Suvvari, T. K., & Thomas, V. (2024). Therapeutic uses of platelet-rich plasma (PRP) in sport injuries–A narrative review. *Journal of Orthopaedic Reports*, *3*(1), 100234.

Peng, G. L. (2019). Platelet-rich plasma for skin rejuvenation: Facts, fiction, and pearls for practice. *Facial Plastic Surgery Clinics of North America*, *27*(3), 331–336. https://doi.org/10.1016/j.fsc.2019.03.004

Pineda-Cortel, M. R., & Cabrera, J. T. (2025). Exploring patients' motivations in using platelet-rich plasma as their primary care therapy for managing knee osteoarthritis: A focus group discussion. *Journal of Primary Care & Community Health*, *16*, 1–9. https://doi.org/10.1177/21501319251323387

Pineda-Cortel, M. R., Suarez, C., & Cabrera, J. T. (2023). Biotherapeutic applications of platelet-rich plasma in regenerative medicine. *Tissue Engineering and Regenerative Medicine*, *20*(5), 681–695. https://doi.org/10.1007/s13770-023-00560-x

Platelet-rich plasma (PRP) in dermatology: Cellular and molecular mechanisms of action. (2023). *Biomedicines*, *12*(1), Article 7. https://doi.org/10.3390/biomedicines12010007

Popescu, M., Iliescu, M., Beiu, C., Popa, L., Mihai, M., Berteanu, M., & Ionescu, A. (2021). Autologous platelet-rich plasma efficacy in the field of regenerative medicine: Product and quality control. *BioMed Research International*, *2021*, Article 4625215.

Pradnyandari, N. K. P. D., & Natasha, R. R. (2022). The role of platelet-rich plasma (PRP) in burn wound healing: A literature-review. *Intisari Sains Medis*, *13*(2), 488–492.

Pritem, A. R., Abraham, V. T., & Krishnagopal, R. (2021). Early clinical and functional outcome of rotator cuff tendinopathy of the shoulder treated with platelet-rich plasma injection. *Malaysian Orthopaedic Journal*, *15*(2), 62–68.

Quicke, D. L. J., Butcher, B. A., & Welton, R. K. (2021). How to use this book. In *Practical R for biologists: An introduction* (pp. 1–6). John Wiley & Sons.

Rachul, C., Rasko, J. E. J., & Caulfield, T. (2017). Implicit hype? Representations of platelet rich plasma in the news media. *PLoS ONE*, *12*(8), Article e0182496. https://doi.org/10.1371/journal.pone.0182496

Rahman, M. S., Rao, P., Abu-Farsakh, H. N., & Thonse, C. (2024). Systematic review of platelet-rich plasma in medical and surgical specialties: Quality, evaluation, evidence, and enforcement. *Journal of Clinical Medicine*, *13*(15), Article 4571. https://doi.org/10.3390/jcm13154571

Raja, A. E., Pigott, T., Pope, D., Tunis, B., & Dougherty, J. (2024). Rehabilitation protocols following platelet-rich plasma injections in the hip. *Current Physical Medicine and Rehabilitation Reports*, *12*(2), 114–121. https://doi.org/10.1007/s40141-024-00436-8

Rodriguez, M., & Mayrovitz, H. N. (2024). The history and current status of platelet-rich plasma therapy in dermatology. *Cureus*, *16*(3), Article e56241. https://doi.org/10.7759/cureus.56241

Rosso, C., Morrey, M., Schär, M., & Grezda, K. (2023). The role of platelet-rich plasma in shoulder pathologies: A critical review of the literature. *EFORT Open Reviews*, *8*(6), 442–453.

Ryder, S., Gnirke, M., Laker, S. R., Hoffmire, C. A., & Comstock, R. (2019). Relationship of overuse injuries and extrascholastic sport participation in high school athletes 2009–2010 through 2015–2016. *PM&R*, *11*(11), 1173–1181. https://doi.org/10.1002/pmrj.12134

Santos, S., Sigurjónsson, Ó., Custódio, C., & Mano, J. (2018). Blood plasma derivatives for tissue engineering and regenerative medicine therapies. *Tissue Engineering Part B: Reviews*, *24*(6), 454–462. https://doi.org/10.1089/ten.teb.2018.0011

Schneider, A., Burr, R., Garbis, N., & Salazar, D. (2018). Platelet-rich plasma and the shoulder: Clinical indications and outcomes. *Current Reviews in Musculoskeletal Medicine*, *11*(4), 593–599. https://doi.org/10.1007/s12178-018-9517-9

Scott, S., Roberts, M., & Chung, E. (2019). Platelet-rich plasma and treatment of erectile dysfunction: Critical review of literature and global trends in platelet-rich plasma clinics. *Sexual Medicine Reviews*, *7*(2), 306–312. https://doi.org/10.1016/j.sxmr.2018.12.005

Scully, D., Naseem, K. M., & Matsakas, A. (2018). Platelet

biology in regenerative medicine of skeletal muscle. *Acta Physiologica, 223*(4), Article e13075.

Sebbagh, P., Hirt-Burri, N., Scaletta, C., & Abdel-Sayed, P. (2023). Process optimization and efficacy assessment of standardized PRP for tendinopathies in sports medicine: Retrospective study of clinical files and GMP manufacturing. *Bioengineering, 10*(4), Article 409. https://doi.org/10.3390/bioengineering10040409

Seyedebrahimi, M. S., Sadeghian, N., Amirpour, M., Jahromi, M., & Hashemi-Beni, B. (2022). Application of platelet-rich plasma (PRP) with different scaffolds in tissue engineering. *Gene, Cell and Tissue, 9*(3), Article e123188. https://doi.org/10.5812/gct-123188

Shimmura, S., Inagaki, E., Hirayama, M., & Hatou, S. (2024). The cornea: An ideal tissue for regenerative medicine. *The Keio Journal of Medicine, 73*(1), 1–10. https://doi.org/10.2302/kjm.2023-0011-RE

Singh, A. S., & Sharun, K. (2023). Prospects of platelet-rich plasma in regenerative medicine. *OBM Transplantation, 7*(2), Article 018. https://doi.org/10.21926/obm.transplant.2302018

Singh, A., Rani, B., & Rawat, S. (2019). Clinical outcome of PRP (Platelet-Rich Plasma) injection in shoulder pain due to rotator cuff disorders. *International Journal of Orthopaedics Sciences, 5*(3), 234–238.

Smid, P., Hart, R., Komzák, M., Paša, L., & Puskeiler, M. (2018). Treatment of partial rotator cuff tears with platelet-rich plasma. *Acta Chirurgiae Orthopaedicae et Traumatologiae Cechoslovaca, 85*(4), 261–266.

Solmaz, I., & Orscelik, A. (2019). Features and clinical effectiveness of the regenerative injection treatments: Prolotherapy and platelet-rich plasma for musculoskeletal pain management. In *Regenerative medicine - Current perspectives and future trends.*

IntechOpen. https://doi.org/10.5772/intechopen.85721

Sulaiman, C., & Rosita, F. (2023). Platelet-rich plasma (PRP) therapy vs minoxidil in men with androgenic alopecia: Systematic review. *International Journal of Social Health*, *2*(6), 342–351. https://doi.org/10.58812/ijsh.v2i06.142

Syed, A. N., Landrum, K., & Ganley, T. J. (2024). Platelet-rich plasma and other injectables in the young athlete. *Orthopedic Clinics of North America*, *55*(2), 215–224.

The use of platelet-rich plasma (PRP) in surgery: Antibiotic effects and post-surgical rehabilitation benefits. (2024). *Journal of Clinical Review & Case Reports*, *9*(3), 88–94. https://doi.org/10.33140/JCRCR.09.03.05

Townsend, C., Von Rickenbach, K. J., & Bailowitz, Z. (2020). Post-procedure protocols following platelet-rich plasma injections for tendinopathy: A systematic review. *PM&R*, *12*(12), 1250–1261. https://doi.org/10.1002/pmrj.12347

van Cauwenberghe, C. (2017). Technology and business trends in regenerative medicine. *Frost & Sullivan Technical Insights*, 1–45.

van Doorn, P. V., Schiphof, D., Rozendaal, R., Ottenheijm, R., van der Lei, J., Bindels, P., & de Schepper, E. D. (2021). The use and safety of corticosteroid injections for shoulder pain in general practice: A retrospective cohort study. *Family Practice*, *38*(5), 604–611. https://doi.org/10.1093/fampra/cmab022

Vincent, K. R., & Sampson, S. (2019). The Orthobiologic Institute 9th annual PRP & regenerative medicine symposium (TOBI 2018): Compendium of abstracts. *Reviews in Pain*, *13*(1), 12–41.

Vinski, N., Vinski, N. C., Sintong, L., & Hardjo, M. (2024). Combination of stem cell & PRP therapy in healthy aging for osteoarthritis. *Journal of World Science*, *3*(2), 180–189. https://doi.org/10.58344/jws.v3i2.564

Wall, C., Johnson, T., Byrnes, J., Crookes, T., & Gill, D. (2023). Chronic shoulder pain. *Australian Journal of General Practice*, *52*(6), 365–371.

Wang, W., Shi, M., Zhou, C., Shi, Z., Cai, X., Lin, T., & Yan, S. (2017). Effectiveness of corticosteroid injections in adhesive capsulitis of shoulder: A meta-analysis. *Medicine*, *96*(28), Article e7445. https://doi.org/10.1097/MD.0000000000007445

Xiao, R. C., Walley, K. C., & DeAngelis, J. P. (2017). Corticosteroid injections for adhesive capsulitis: A review. *Clinical Journal of Sport Medicine*, *27*(3), 314–320. https://doi.org/10.1097/JSM.0000000000000348

Xu, Y., Li, T., Wang, L., Yao, L., & Li, J. (2024). Platelet-rich plasma has better results for long-term functional improvement and pain relief for lateral epicondylitis: A systematic review and meta-analysis of randomized controlled trials. *The American Journal of Sports Medicine*, *52*(4), 1085–1096. https://doi.org/10.1177/03635465231213087

Yonai, Y., Lever, L., Ben Natan, M., Shteinfeld, Y., Seroguon, Y., & Berkovich, Y. (2022). Treatment of rotator cuff disease with platelet-rich plasma injections. *Harefuah*, *161*(8), 492–496.

Zhang, W. B., Ma, Y. L., Lu, F. L., Guo, H. R., & Song, H. (2024). The clinical efficacy and safety of platelet-rich plasma on frozen shoulder: A systematic review and meta-analysis of randomized controlled trials. *BMC Musculoskeletal Disorders*, *25*(1), Article 534. https://doi.org/10.1186/s12891-024-07629-1

CHAPTER 2

Common Shoulder Conditions & PRP Treatment Areas

Author: David Espinoza

Shoulder Anatomy Overview

The shoulder is one of the most complex structures in the human body. It is woven together in a unique construct of bone, ligament, and myotendinous anatomy. The upper arm bone, known as the humerus, forms the humeral head, which then articulates with the glenoid bone from the scapula to form the glenohumeral joint. Most refer to this as the 'shoulder joint' (Figure 2.1). Just above that, the clavicle comes across the top of the glenohumeral joint and articulates with the coracoid of the scapula as well as the acromion of the scapula, creating the acromioclavicular joint, also known as the 'AC' joint (Figure 2.1). Seeing as the glenohumeral joint is shaped somewhat like a golf ball sitting on a tee, it allows for great mobility of the shoulder, more than any other joint, but with the increased mobility comes increased instability of that joint. Every bone that articulates and forms a joint with another has a lining called cartilage. To help with this mobile structure, there are static stabilizers called ligaments that surround the shoulder to help secure the bones in place, including the glenohumeral ligaments, transverse humeral ligament, coracohumeral ligament, coracoacromial ligament, acromioclavicular ligament, and coracoclavicular ligaments (Figure 2.2).

Embedded between the glenoid bone and the humeral head is an extension of cartilage known as the labrum, which also helps support the humeral head within the glenoid. The rotator cuff muscles and tendons also play a very important role as dynamic stabilizers for the shoulder, but also allow for the wide range of motion with the joint that includes the supraspinatus, infraspinatus, teres minor, and the subscapularis (Figure 2.3). Just above the rotator cuff tendons, underneath the acromion, sits the subacromial bursa, which is a sack of fluid that is present to reduce friction between the rotator cuff tendons and the acromion bone. The surrounding biceps tendon, deltoid, trapezius, rhomboids, latissimus dorsi, and pectoral muscles are also supporting actors that help give the shoulder stability and strength to allow for the various capabilities of the shoulder joint. It is crucial to understand this unique anatomy when it comes to the treatment of shoulder pathology because whether it be the AC joint, the supraspinatus tendon, or the glenohumeral ligament that has the problem, all that will register to the patient is that "my shoulder hurts!" Ensuring proper treatment for the proper problem and pathology with the proper solution is vital to optimizing patient outcomes as a whole, especially when it comes to treatment with orthobiologics.

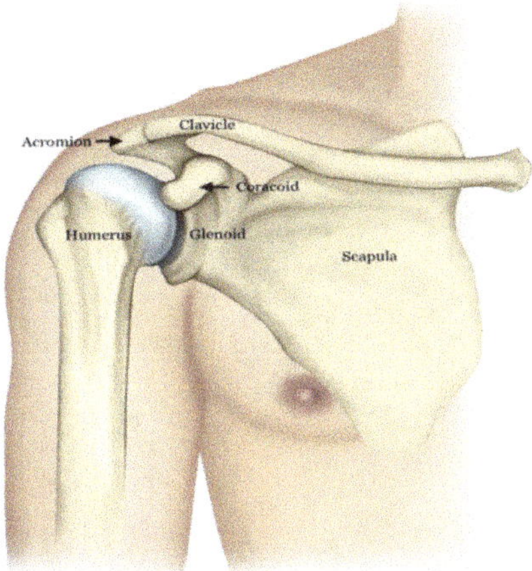

Figure 2.1 Basic Bony Anatomy of the Shoulder Joint

This illustration demonstrates the primary osseous structures of the shoulder, including the clavicle, acromion, coracoid process, scapula, glenoid, and proximal humerus. Together, these structures form the glenohumeral joint and surrounding shoulder girdle, providing the foundation for shoulder mobility, stability, and upper extremity function.

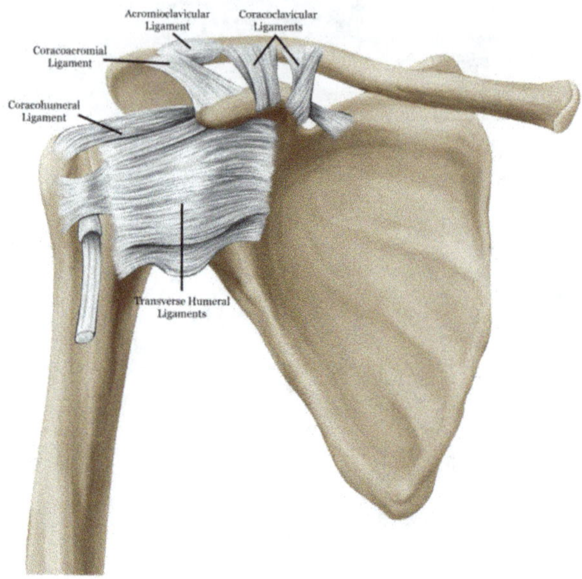

Figure 2.2 Major Static Stabilizing Ligaments of the Shoulder Complex

This illustration depicts the principal ligamentous structures of the shoulder, including the acromioclavicular ligament, coracoclavicular ligaments, coracoacromial ligament, coracohumeral ligament, and transverse humeral ligament. These ligaments provide static stability to the shoulder girdle, helping maintain joint alignment while supporting normal shoulder motion and function.

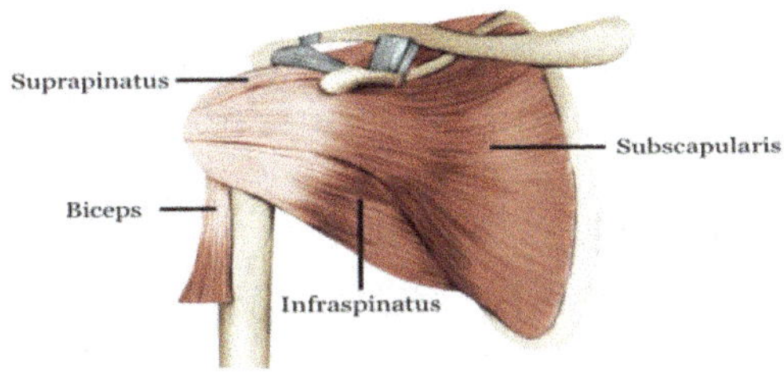

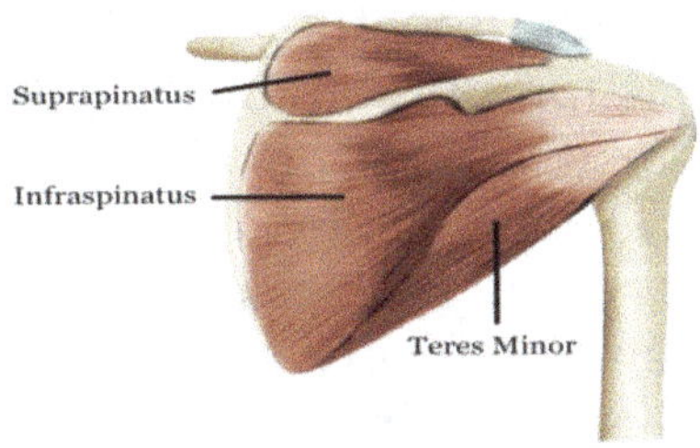

Figure 2.3 Rotator Cuff Musculature and the Long Head of the Biceps Tendon

This illustration depicts the four muscles of the rotator cuff—supraspinatus, infraspinatus, teres minor, and subscapularis—as well as the long head of the biceps tendon. Together, these structures provide dynamic stability to the glenohumeral joint while facilitating shoulder motion, including elevation, rotation, and functional upper extremity activities.

Rotator Cuff Injuries

The four rotator cuff muscles and tendons that support the shoulder are vital to the joint's stability and function. Rotator cuff tendon pathology can result from sudden acute injuries and from chronic repetitive use. Acute damage to the tendons can result from sudden traumatic injuries such as a fall or a direct blow to the shoulder. Acute damage can also occur suddenly when attempting to lift a heavy weight while the muscle and tendon are in a stretched position. Chronic disease of the rotator cuff tendons can develop over time as a result of repetitive use. This can lead to long-term inflammation of the tendons, a condition known as tendinosis. When tendinosis occurs, there is microdamage to the tendon fibers which leads to a loss of elasticity and subsequent tendon pathology. This is often also referred to as tendinopathy. Additionally, chronic rotator cuff tendon pathology can occur as a result of mechanical rubbing of the tendon from a bone spur off of the acromion. Postural deficits can also lead to a situation where the rotator cuff is more at risk of mechanical structural damage from surrounding bony spurs. Finally, general overall tendon health can be affected by smoking and by cardiovascular disease and diabetes, which tendon to make the tendons more susceptible to chronic damage.

Rotator cuff injuries are fairly common, especially as people age. Studies have shown that they can affect approximately 20 to 30% of the general population. Rotator cuff tears can be partial-thickness or full-thickness tears. Partial-thickness rotator cuff tears are further classified as low-grade, mid-grade or high-grade, depending on the width and length of the tear. These partial-thickness rotator cuff tears cause pain that can radiate around the entire shoulder and into the upper part of the arm. The pain is often worse at night and with certain movements. Patients can have well-maintained mobility in the setting of a partial rotator cuff tear, although weakness can be perceived. By contrast, full-thickness, rotator cuff tears can occur when the entirety of the tendon insertion onto the bone becomes detached or from an extension of a partial-thickness tear. These types of tears typically lead to a loss of function. Often, because the anchor point of the tendon on the bone has fully torn, there will be significant weakness and limitations in range of motion. During physical examination, certain maneuvers can clue in the physician on the severity of the tear. But typically, advanced imaging, such as magnetic resonance imaging (MRI) or diagnostic musculoskeletal ultrasound, is needed to confirm the suspected pathology.

PRP can be used to treat rotator cuff tendinosis/tendinopathy as well as rotator cuff tears. It is important to distinguish between partial versus full-thickness rotator cuff tears when considering these regenerative Ortho biologic options, since studies have indicated the partial-thickness tears (even large ones) may benefit and do quite well with PRP and may help prevent the progression to full-thickness tears. By contrast, so far, the evidence for PRP and full-thickness tears is less robust. Tendinopathy and tendinosis of the rotator cuff tendons are conditions that also respond very well to PRP. The immunomodulatory cascade can lead to stimulation of collagen remodeling within the tendon to allow for improved elasticity and function over the long-term.

There are numerous research articles ranging from level 1 to level 4 evidence that demonstrate that PRP is beneficial in the short and long-term with regard to pain and function when it comes to rotator cuff partial tears as well as rotator cuff tendinopathy. The research does note issues with the variability of PRP study methodology since PRP remains non-standardized. However, even with this variation, there is still strong mounting evidence that demonstrates that PRP can be effective at treating rotator cuff injuries and tendinopathy when compared to other conservative and traditional treatment modalities.

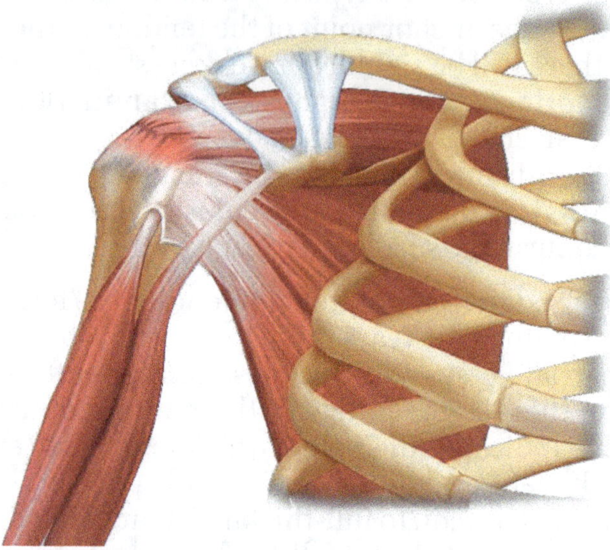

Figure 2.4 Partial-Thickness Supraspinatus Tear of the Rotator Cuff

This illustration demonstrates a partial-thickness tear of the supraspinatus tendon at its insertion on the greater tuberosity of the humerus. The image highlights the close relationship between the rotator cuff tendons, the long head of the biceps tendon, and the overlying acromial structures. Partial-thickness tears commonly develop as a result of tendon degeneration, repetitive overhead activity, mechanical impingement, or acute injury and may contribute to shoulder pain, weakness, and dysfunction.

Shoulder Osteoarthritis (Glenohumeral and Acromioclavicular Joint)

Osteoarthritis (OA) of the shoulder is another condition that can be quite limiting once the arthritis advances in degree and severity. Patients will typically wake up in the mornings with stiffness in the shoulder area, and they feel it will take a little while for the stiffness to improve, along with the range of motion, once they get up. Some will have a lull in the pain, but then, as the shoulder is used throughout the day, the pain becomes worse, and they will tend to have even more pain as they lie down to rest at day's end. Those suffering from glenohumeral joint OA tend to localize pain as a deep-seated discomfort in the shoulder area, either in the front or back of the shoulder. However, those suffering from acromioclavicular joint OA tend to be very pinpoint with localizing pain in the top portion of the shoulder area. Pain is typically worse when lying on their side or reaching overhead or across their body to the opposite side. Exam findings, including tenderness to palpation in the area of the joint space and provocative maneuvers, can elicit pain. There may also be a limited range of motion due to the mechanical block of the bones from arthritis, deteriorating the joint space itself. X-ray findings, along with history and physical exam, are sufficient to make the diagnosis of osteoarthritis.

The traditional treatment for osteoarthritis of the shoulder has included NSAIDs (nonsteroidal anti-inflammatory drugs), physical therapy, topical creams, and corticosteroids. However, mounting evidence in studies indicates that the correct formulation and dosage of PRP can be superior in both short-term and long-term effects compared to more traditional modalities of treatment. The high-dose platelets delivered to the affected joint would initiate a cascade of immunomodulatory effects that would provide an anti-inflammatory environment in the joint, but just as importantly, help promote a healing response of the cartilage layer in the joint, attempting to preserve the joint over the long run. It is prudent to be accurate with the diagnosis as both the glenohumeral and acromioclavicular joints are encased in their own capsule of tissue, and an injection would need to be accurate and pinpoint in order for patients to have the optimal outcome with the desired effects from the PRP procedure. The severity of the arthritis and narrowing of the joint space can make these injections challenging, which emphasizes the use of ultrasound or fluoroscopic image guidance in order to deliver injections into these joints.

Research studies indicate that patients with mild to moderate osteoarthritis of the shoulder demonstrated statistically significant improvement in pain and function with PRP injections for shoulder OA.

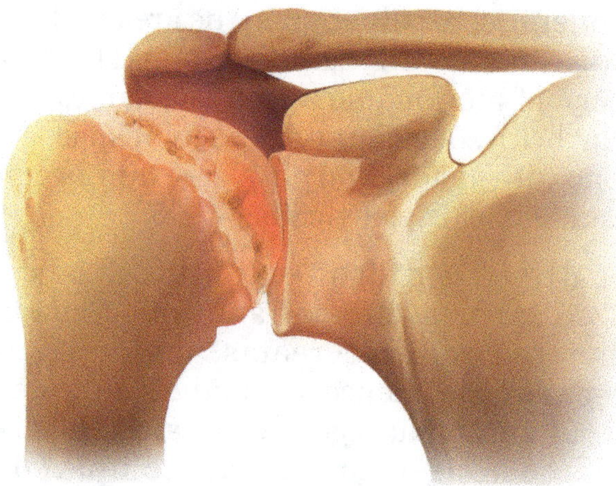

Figure 2.5 Glenohumeral Osteoarthritis of the Shoulder Joint

This illustration depicts osteoarthritis of the glenohumeral joint, characterized by progressive cartilage loss, joint space narrowing, subchondral bone remodeling, and osteophyte (bone spur) formation. As the protective cartilage wears away, increased bone-on-bone contact may occur, leading to pain, stiffness, crepitus, reduced range of motion, and functional limitations. Glenohumeral osteoarthritis is a common cause of chronic shoulder pain, particularly in older adults and individuals with a history of prior shoulder injury or surgery.

Bursitis & Chronic Inflammation

Subacromial bursitis accounts for about 0.4% of all primary care visits and is a common cause of shoulder pain in general. The pain is typically sharp and will limit the range of motion of the shoulder due to the pain with motion. There is also pain when lying on the side of the shoulder. The bursa is there to help reduce friction between the rotator cuff tendons and surrounding bony structures, particularly the acromion and underneath the acromioclavicular joint. The bursa may become inflamed with repetitive overhead activity and usage, especially if there is underlying rotator cuff tendinopathy, osteoarthritic changes involving the acromioclavicular joint, and osteophyte formations, or even in the setting of a down-sloping acromion that could predispose the bursa to increased friction. Direct trauma to the shoulder could also lead to bursitis and chronic inflammation.

Through the release of specific cytokine proteins, platelet-derived growth factors, and pro-inflammatory markers in the blood, PRP has the ability to re-initiate the body's healing potential, which can break chronic inflammatory cycles—this allows for PRP to have an anti-inflammatory effect on persistent and chronic bursitis by down-regulating the inflammatory cytokine proteins that keep propagating the inflammation in the bursa. Research has also demonstrated improved outcomes compared to steroid injections for subacromial bursitis over a 3–6-month period as well. Chronic biceps tenosynovitis in the shoulder may also be amenable to treatment with PRP, given the persistent inflammation with that disease process as well.

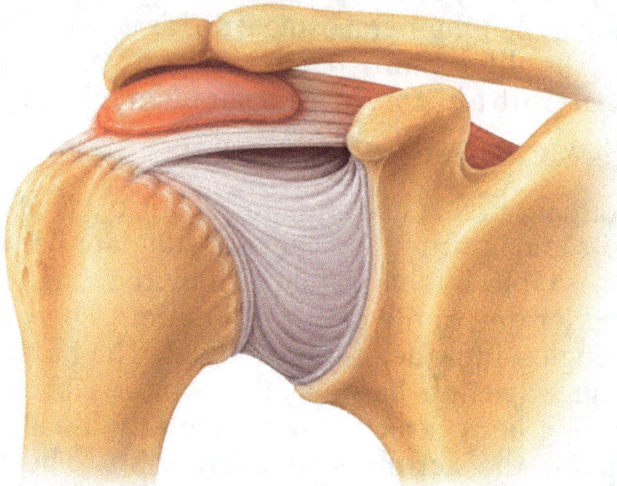

Figure 2.6 Subacromial Bursitis of the Shoulder

This illustration demonstrates inflammation and distention of the subacromial bursa located between the rotator cuff tendons and the undersurface of the acromion. Enlargement of the bursa may reduce the available subacromial space, contributing to pain, impingement symptoms, and discomfort during overhead shoulder activities.

Labral Tears & Shoulder Instability

The glenoid labrum within the glenohumeral joint is an extension of fibrocartilage that helps provide stability as it coats the glenoid and interacts directly with the humeral head. This structure also protects the joint space, and damage to it could potentially lead to long-term degradation of the shoulder joint and subsequent osteoarthritis. Labral damage can occur from trauma such as a fall or a sports injury. It can also occur due to repetitive overuse. Labral tears are also common in people with hyperligamentous laxity, excessive range of motion, and chronic instability. The surrounding structures, including the ligaments as well as the rotator cuff, are important in helping the labrum stabilize the joint, and should those structures not do their jobs, then the labrum must take the brunt of stabilizing the joint, which can lead to more damage over time. Injury to the labrum is described by location and complexity of the tear, and if other associated structures are included, such as the biceps tendon. Labral tear locations are localized with reference to hands on a clock face, with 12:00 being on top, 3:00 in front, 6:00 at the bottom, and 9:00 in the back of the shoulder joint. Some labral tears are very severe and can contribute to chronic dislocations of the shoulder. In these cases, surgical consultation is warranted. Patients will tend to feel pain either in the front, top, or back part of the shoulder that is worse with certain positions and certain loads on the shoulder joint. On examination, there are multiple special tests that would help the clinician discern if there is concern for labrum damage or shoulder instability. Advanced imaging with an MRI or MR arthrogram is typically necessary to assess the full extent of the labral damage.

PRP and its disease-modifying effects with immunomodulation and cartilage preservation may be an effective treatment for labral damage and ligament instability of the shoulder joint, particularly when coupled with physical therapy that is geared toward shoulder and scapular stabilization. In cases where surgery is required, studies have shown improved recovery, improved healing, and improved functional outcomes when PRP is performed at 12 months post-operatively.

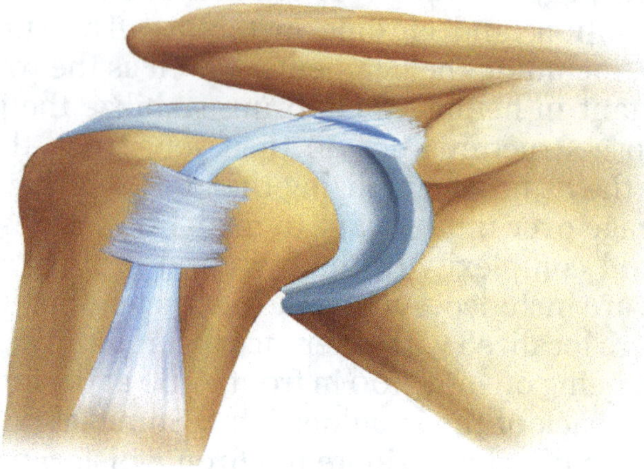

Figure 2.7 Labral Tear at the Biceps-Labral Anchor Complex

This illustration demonstrates a tear of the superior glenoid labrum at the attachment site of the long head of the biceps tendon, commonly referred to as the biceps-labral anchor. Injuries in this region may occur as a result of repetitive overhead activity, traction forces, shoulder instability, or acute trauma. Labral tears at the biceps-labral anchor can contribute to shoulder pain, clicking, catching, loss of function, and difficulty with overhead or athletic activities.

Frozen Shoulder (Adhesive Capsulitis)

The condition of Adhesive Capsulitis, also known as Frozen Shoulder, is a very painful and functionally limiting shoulder pathology that affects approximately 2%–5% of the population. Frozen Shoulder affects middle-aged individuals and more commonly affects women and those with endocrine disorders such as diabetes mellitus and thyroid disorders. It is believed that these disorders may increase the body's inflammatory state and fibrotic responses; the exact cause of frozen shoulder remains unknown. When frozen shoulder occurs, there is an interplay between the overall inflammation and the increased fibrotic response, thus leading to the formation of adhesions within the shoulder capsule, which leads to increased pain and limited range of motion in nearly all directions of the shoulder. The synovial lining of the joint will thicken due to the inflammatory response, and the capsule itself becomes thickened with the increased fibrous tissue as well. Initially, at times, patients may not have too much pain, but then over weeks to months, the pain becomes so debilitating that it will nearly stop people from being functional altogether. An exam typically entails a patient unable or not willing to move their shoulder, particularly with flexion, abduction, and external rotation. The hallmark of frozen shoulder is a limitation in both passive and active range of motion that is observed in all planes of motion, in the absence of significant shoulder arthritis. Imaging with an MRI may show capsular thickening, thickened coracohumeral ligament, rotator interval synovitis, and/or a decrease in size of the axillary pouch. Correct diagnosis is prudent as prognosis is improved when the condition is treated sooner rather than later, initially with anti-inflammatories, physical therapy, and/or injections. Approximately 80% of patients will regain a full range of motion and function, but unfortunately, 10%–20% may end up with residual stiffness or pain. The condition occurs in 3 distinct stages: the initial phase is the "freezing" where people feel disabling pain along with limited range of motion and can last from 2 to 9 months in duration; this is followed by the intermediate "frozen" stage where the pain will subside some but there is still a fair amount of limited motion due to the capsule thickening and can last from 4–12 months. The third and final phase is the thawing phase, where a gradual reduction in pain and slow improvement in range of motion occur. This phase can take 18 months to three years for full resolution. Traditionally, corticosteroid injections have been part of the treatment algorithm, but they could lead to adverse effects. In severe cases, surgery is warranted with manipulation under anesthesia and capsular release.

PRP has been studied in the treatment of frozen shoulder. Large systematic literature reviews indicate that PRP improves short-term and long-term outcomes in the disease process. Furthermore, PRP injections outperformed corticosteroid injections at 12 weeks after treatment. This is very promising since there exists a high correlation between frozen shoulder and diabetes, and corticosteroid injections could adversely affect blood sugars in a diabetic patient. The cascade of inflammatory markers and proteins initiated by a PRP injection can have a direct effect on each of the three phases in the disease process and can subsequently have an overall anti-inflammatory response with decreased fibrotic changes in the collagen within the capsule itself. Overall, PRP is an effective form of treatment at each stage of Adhesive Capsulitis that is capable of producing lasting effects.

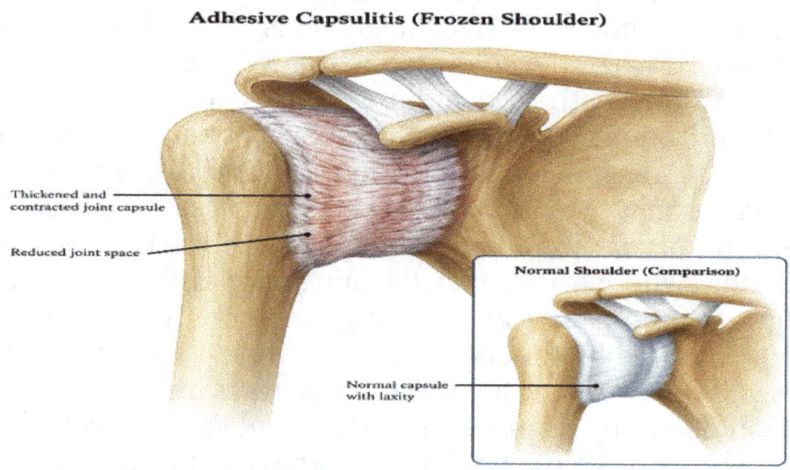

Figure 2.8 Adhesive Capsulitis (Frozen Shoulder): Capsular Thickening and Contracture

This illustration demonstrates adhesive capsulitis, commonly known as frozen shoulder, characterized by thickening, inflammation, and contracture of the glenohumeral joint capsule. These pathologic changes lead to reduced capsular volume, restricted joint motion, pain, and progressive loss of shoulder mobility. The inset comparison highlights the difference between a normal, compliant joint capsule and the contracted capsule seen in adhesive capsulitis.

Table 2.1 Summary Table of PRP Studies for Common Shoulder Conditions

Condition Treated	Study Author	Year	Number of Patients	Outcomes	Key Takeaways
Adhesive Capsulitis	Singh et al.	2025	~70	VAS, SPADI, ROM (1-year)	PRP showed more durable improvement than steroids
Adhesive Capsulitis	Somisetty et al.	2023	60	VAS, SPADI, ROM	PRP is superior at mid–late follow-up
Adhesive Capsulitis	Gupta et al.	2022	60	Pain, DASH, ROM	Greater improvement at 12 weeks with PRP
Adhesive Capsulitis	Karabaş et al.	2019	50	VAS, Constant, ROM	Progressive improvement over time
Adhesive Capsulitis	Cureus RCT	2021	40	VAS, SPADI	PRP is longer-lasting than steroids
Rotator Cuff Tendinopathy	Rossi et al.	2024	80	VAS, Constant, ASES	More sustained benefit with PRP
Partial Rotator Cuff Tear	Guity et al.	2025	64	VAS, Constant	Steroid faster early relief
Rotator Cuff Repair (Surgical)	Rossi et al.	2024	90	MRI retear rate, PROMs	Lower retear rate with LP-PRP
Rotator Cuff Repair (Surgical)	Yao et al.	2024	120	Healing rate, PROMs	LP-PRP is superior to LR-PRP
Glenohumeral OA	Kirschner et al.	2022	70	VAS, ASES, WOOS	PRP is similar to HA

Key Takeaways

As we have shown, the functioning of the shoulder joint is a complex interaction of many different structures. Pain in the shoulder can arise from any number of conditions. When considering PRP, it is essential to use the history and physical exam, as well as any confirmatory imaging, when making an accurate diagnosis. Successful outcomes in the treatment of the shoulder structures with PRP depend on appropriate diagnosis of the affected structure, and on image-guided targeting of the platelet injection to that affected tissue. Based on studies and research, partial rotator cuff tears, shoulder joint osteoarthritis, ligament instability, labral tears, and adhesive capsulitis all demonstrate reliable responses when treated with PRP, so long as the proper dosage and proper technique are used for PRP treatment. That is why it is prudent and necessary to consult with a qualified physician to ensure that the shoulder pain being experienced will, in fact, improve and respond to PRP. Patients should feel confident that the correct problem is being addressed, and they should have a good understanding of how their condition is going to be treated with the procedure itself. Qualified consultation is valuable so that patients may better understand all that is going to happen on the PRP procedure day itself.

Bibliography

Azharuddin, S., Gahlot, N., Elhence, A., Garg, P., Mandal, S., & Saxena, S. (2025). Improved healing and functional outcome is seen at 12 months after injecting leukocyte rich-PRP in arthroscopically repaired labrum: A case-control study. *Shoulder & Elbow, 17*(1), 45–53. https://doi.org/10.1177/17585732251319259

Barman, A., Mukherjee, S., Sahoo, J., Maiti, R., Rao, B. P., Sinha, M. K., Sahoo, D., Tripathy, S. K., Patro, B. K., & Bag, N. D. (2019). Single intra-articular platelet-rich plasma versus corticosteroid injections in the treatment of adhesive capsulitis of the shoulder: A cohort study. *American Journal of Physical Medicine & Rehabilitation, 98*(7), 549–557. https://doi.org/10.1097/PHM.0000000000001144

Bhan, K., & Singh, B. (2022). Efficacy of platelet-rich plasma injection in the management of rotator cuff tendinopathy: A review of the current literature. *Cureus, 14*(6), Article e26103. https://doi.org/10.7759/cureus.26103

Blanchard, E., Harvi, J., Vasudevan, J., & Swanson, R. L., 2nd. (2023). Platelet-rich plasma for adhesive capsulitis: A systematic review. *Cureus, 15*(10), Article e46580. https://doi.org/10.7759/cureus.46580

Chen, X., Jones, I. A., Park, C., & Vangsness, C. T. (2017). The efficacy of platelet-rich plasma on tendon and ligament healing: A systematic review and meta-analysis with bias assessment. *The American Journal of Sports Medicine, 46*(8), 2020–2032. https://doi.org/10.1177/0363546517743746

Chen, X., Jones, I. A., Togashi, R., Park, C., & Vangsness, C. T. (2019). Use of platelet-rich plasma for the improvement of pain and function in rotator cuff tears:

A systematic review and meta-analysis with bias assessment. *The American Journal of Sports Medicine*, *48*(8), 2028–2041. https://doi.org/10.1177/0363546519881423

Cole, B. J., Cotter, E. J., Wang, K. C., & Davey, A. (2017). Patient understanding, expectations, and satisfaction regarding rotator cuff injuries and surgical management. *Arthroscopy: The Journal of Arthroscopic & Related Surgery*, *33*(8), 1603–1606. https://doi.org/10.1016/j.arthro.2017.03.017

Faruqi, T., & Rizvi, T. J. (2023). *Subacromial bursitis*. StatPearls Publishing. https://www.ncbi.nlm.nih.gov/books/NBK541096/

Hudgens, J. L., Sugg, K. B., Grekin, J. A., Gumucio, J. P., Bedi, A., & Mendias, C. L. (2016). Platelet-rich plasma activates proinflammatory signaling pathways and induces oxidative stress in tendon fibroblasts. *The American Journal of Sports Medicine*, *44*(8), 1931–1940. https://doi.org/10.1177/0363546516637176

Khodary, M. S. E., et al. (2024). Effect of leukocyte-rich PRP on interstitial or partial tear of rotator cuff of shoulder. *International Journal of Life Sciences Biotechnology and Pharma Research*, *13*(1), 112–120.

Li, D., St Angelo, J. M., & Taqi, M. (2025). *Adhesive capsulitis (frozen shoulder)*. StatPearls Publishing. https://www.ncbi.nlm.nih.gov/books/NBK532955/

Prodromos, C. C., Finkle, S., Prodromos, A., et al. (2021). Treatment of rotator cuff tears with platelet rich plasma: A prospective study with 2 year follow-up. *BMC Musculoskeletal Disorders*, *22*, Article 499. https://doi.org/10.1186/s12891-021-04288-4

Rathod, V., Shrivastav, S., & Gharpinde, M. R. (2024). Platelet-rich plasma therapy for rotator cuff injuries: A comprehensive review of current evidence and future directions. *Cureus*, *16*(9), Article e70042. https://doi.org/10.7759/cureus.70042

Saif, D. S., Serag, D. M., & El Tabl, M. A. (2019). Comparative study between platelet-rich plasma injection and steroid injection in mild–moderate shoulder osteoarthritis and their relation to quality of life. *Egyptian Rheumatology and Rehabilitation*, *46*, 55–61.

Shams, A., El-Sayed, M., Gamal, O., et al. (2016). Subacromial injection of autologous platelet-rich plasma versus corticosteroid for the treatment of symptomatic partial rotator cuff tears. *European Journal of Orthopaedic Surgery & Traumatology*, *26*, 837–842. https://doi.org/10.1007/s00590-016-1826-3

Zhu, P., Wang, Z., Li, H., & Cai, Y. (2022). Platelet-rich plasma injection in non-operative treatment of partial-thickness rotator cuff tears: A systematic review and meta-analysis. *Journal of Rehabilitation Medicine*, *54*, Article jrm00312. https://doi.org/10.2340/jrm.v54.1434

CHAPTER 3

Understanding the Hard Science of PRP

Authors: Peter A. Everts, L. Podesta, Andre van Zundert & José Fabio Lana

Introduction

Platelet-Rich plasma (PRP), the platelet-enriched fraction of autologous blood, has been applied in clinical practice for over 30 years and is increasingly recognized as a key orthobiological preparation in regenerative medicine. Its diverse mix of platelets and leukocytes offers therapeutic potential for musculoskeletal (MSK) disorders, leveraging numerous platelet-derived growth factors (PGFs) and many bioactive molecules originating from platelets and other PRP constituents to drive inflammation control, angiogenesis, painkilling, and ultimately functional tissue repair.

Despite encouraging patient outcomes, inconsistencies persist in PRP therapy, stemming from variabilities across 50 identified commercial PRP systems, diverse preparation protocols, and a lack of standardized bioformulation reporting.

These variations lead to significant differences in PRP composition, including platelet concentration, growth factor levels, and cellular content. For instance, studies have shown that centrifugation parameters can significantly impact fibrin structure, cellular distribution, and biomolecular content of PRP. Additionally, the absence of mandatory reporting requirements for key parameters such as platelet, white blood cell, and red blood cell concentrations hinders reproducibility and cross-study comparisons. Recent advances have refined the understanding of platelet granular biology, cell membrane receptor function, and immune modulation via both innate and adaptive pathways. Research now highlights PRP's influence on mesenchymal stem cell (MSC) activity, paracrine signaling, and the regenerative microenvironment. This chapter summarizes current insights into PRP preparation, dosing, and composition; cellular and molecular mechanisms; analgesic effects; drug interactions; and strategies for integrating PRP into comprehensive rehabilitation protocols. By dissecting the granular biology and immunomodulatory pathways, this chapter addresses these critical variabilities, moving beyond mere acknowledgement of the issue to offer a deeper understanding towards industry-wide standardization, thereby fulfilling a crucial research gap.

The Rationale for Platelet-Rich Plasma Therapies

PRP applications have gained widespread adoption across multiple medical specialties due to their potential to enhance functional tissue repair. The therapeutic premise is that delivering concentrated platelets to an injury site triggers the release of growth factors, cytokines, lysosomal enzymes, and adhesion proteins, initiating the hemostatic cascade, stimulating connective tissue synthesis, and promoting revascularization. The accompanying platelet-poor plasma (PPP) fraction also contains plasma proteins such as fibrinogen, prothrombin, and fibronectin, which contribute to the non-platelet contributing repair processes. PRP can potentially induce a supraphysiological surge of growth factors, accelerating healing in acute injuries and reactivating stalled repair processes in chronic pathological and tissue-specific conditions. Throughout tissue healing, a diverse array of bioactive molecules and signaling pathways, including endocrine, paracrine, autocrine, and intracrine mechanisms, drive essential cell functions. Key advantages of PRP include its autologous origin, favorable safety profile, and the adaptability of modern preparation systems that enable broad clinical use. However, the absence of standardized regulations for PRP formulation leads to wide variability in platelet concentration, leukocyte content, red blood cell contamination, and growth factor levels, making reproducibility and outcome consistency an ongoing challenge.

PRP: A Myriad of Reparative Proteins and Molecular Stimulators and Actors

Platelets are essential for primary hemostasis and play a significant role in regulating angiogenesis, inflammation, and immunomodulation. Angiogenic stimulators are released from various sources, including platelets, endothelial cells, fibroblasts, smooth muscle cells, leukocytes, and inflammatory cells. Platelets are known to release angiogenic regulatory proteins, platelet-derived growth factors (PDGFs), cytokines, and chemokines, which are crucial for angiogenesis, as demonstrated in numerous *in vitro* and animal studies.

Platelet Dosing and Bioformulation in Angiogenesis Regulation

Although the role of platelets in angiogenesis is well-established, the development of tissue-specific PRP formulations with customized platelet doses for chronic pathoanatomic conditions remains underexplored. The general belief that PRP is a "one-size-fits-all" solution for angiogenesis limits its potential for optimizing tissue repair. The variability in PRP therapy outcomes can be attributed to the frequent use of single-spin PRP tubes with low platelet capture rates. Consequently, the platelet concentration and leukocyte presence in PRP significantly influence tissue microvasculature restoration and repair mechanisms, which are critical for improving patient outcomes.

Platelets

Platelets are small, anucleate discoid blood cells, measuring 1–3 μm, produced by megakaryocytes in the red bone marrow and released into the circulation in a resting state. Adult platelet counts range from 150 to 350 × 10^6/mL. Platelets contain extracellular glycoprotein receptors, adhesion molecules, and three intra-platelet structures: alpha-granules, dense granules, and lysosomes, each with specific cellular and molecular contents. Platelets stimulate cell proliferation, the synthesis of mesenchymal and neurotrophic factors, chemotactic migration, immunomodulation, and angiogenesis. Giusti and colleagues identified that a platelet concentration of 1.5 × 10^6 platelets/μL is optimal for stimulating tissue repair and inducing angiogenesis through endothelial cells, while higher platelet concentrations may reduce angiogenic capacity in follicular and perifollicular angiogenesis.

Platelet Granules

Early clinical interest in PRP focused on α-granules, which contain coagulation factors, abundant platelet-derived growth factors (PDGFs), and angiogenesis regulators, but only minimal pro-thrombotic activity. These granules also store less well-known chemokines and cytokines—such as platelet factor 4 (PF4), pro-platelet basic protein, P-selectin (an integrin activator), and RANTES (Regulated upon Activation, Normal T Cell Expressed and Presumably Secreted)—which recruit and activate immune cells or stimulate endothelial inflammation (Figure 3.1).

Dense granules contain bioactive molecules, including ADP, serotonin, polyphosphates, histamine, and epinephrine, which not only influence platelet activation and thrombus formation but also exert significant immune-modulating effects. For example:

- Platelet ADP binds to P2Y12 receptors on dendritic cells (DCs), enhancing antigen uptake.
- Platelet ATP signals via P2X7 receptors on T cells, promoting differentiation of CD4 T-helper cells into pro-inflammatory Th17 cells.
- Glutamate can stimulate T-cell migration, while serotonin promotes monocyte differentiation into DCs.

In PRP, these dense platelet granule-derived molecules are present at enriched levels, contributing substantially to innate and adaptive immune regulation.

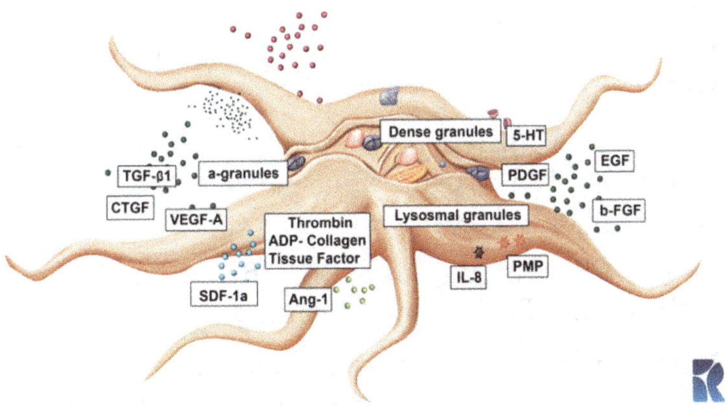

Figure 3.1 Graphical Presentation and Activated Platelets

Normally, in PRP, platelets are in a resting, nonactivated state. Upon (tissue) activation, platelets change their shape with the development of pseudopods to promote platelet aggregation and the subsequent release of their granular content through the open canalicular system.

PGF binds to specific cell membrane receptors.

After PRP has been applied to tissues, a PRP clot will develop as a result of tissue factor activation. Subsequently, the clot will start to retract, and the PRP clot will lyse, with the degranulation of the granular platelet content, PGFs, and other molecules and cytokines, which will be deposited in the extracellular matrix of the injected tissue structures.

The entire process of platelet receptor binding in the context of PRP application involves several key steps and can be summarized as follows:

1. **Growth factor deposition**: After PRP application, platelets degranulate and release growth factors into the extracellular matrix.
2. **Matrix degradation**: Over time, the extracellular matrix degrades, releasing the deposited growth factors.
3. **Ligand-receptor interaction**: Released growth factors bind to tyrosine kinase receptors (TKRs) on the surface of target tissue cells.
4. **Receptor activation**: Binding of growth factors activates the TKRs, which span the cell membrane.
5. **Intracellular signaling**: Activated TKRs trigger intracellular signaling cascades by interacting with cytoplasmic messenger proteins.

6. **Nuclear signaling**: Activated messenger proteins enter the cell nucleus and influence gene expression related to cell division and tissue repair.
7. **Biological response**: This leads to transcription of mRNA and subsequent biological responses that promote tissue repair and regeneration.

Additionally, PGFs can act in three modes:

1. **Paracrine**: Affecting nearby cells of different types
2. **Autocrine**: Affecting the cell that produced them
3. **Endocrine**: Affecting distant cells of different types

Growth factors in platelet-rich plasma (PRP) exhibit versatile modes of action, enabling them to influence various cell types across different tissue structures and pathologies. This multifaceted capability and versatility of growth factors allow PRP to trigger a cascade of cellular responses, potentially leading to diverse biological and reparative effects across multiple (pathological) biological systems.

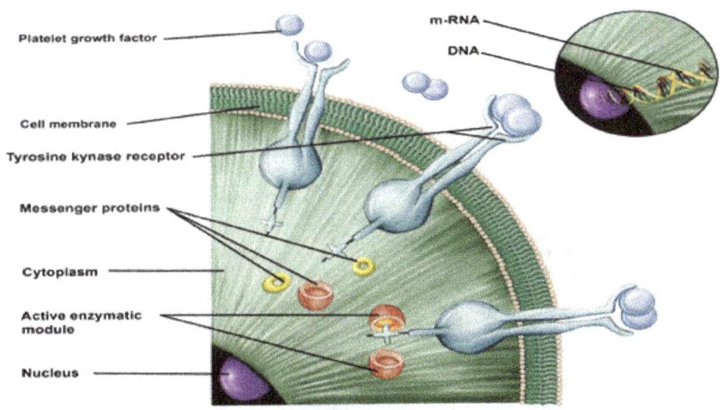

Figure 3.2 Cellular Signaling Pathways Activated by Platelet Growth Factors

Diagram showing the mechanism by which specific platelet-derived growth factors (PGFs) bind to their corresponding receptors on the target cell membrane, initiating intracellular signaling cascades. These signaling events regulate cellular functions such as proliferation, migration, differentiation, extracellular matrix production, and tissue repair within the treated tissue.

Table 3.1 Partial List of PRP-platelet Structures with their Specific Components

Structure	Key Content	Main Functions
α-granules	*Growth Factors:* PDGF (AA-BB-AB-CC), VEGF, TGF (α-β), FGF (a-b), EGF, CTGF	Growth factor-based regulation of tissue repair via cell proliferation, differentiation, mitogenesis, chemotaxis, and epithelial repair.
	Adhesive Proteins: Fibronectin, vitronectin, vWF fibrinogen, P-selectin, integrins αIIbβ, Phosphatidylserine	Platelet aggregation, platelet-endothelial cell interaction, and thrombus formation.
	Coagulation Factors: Factors IV, XI, XIII, plasminogen, plasmin, antithrombin, Tissue Factor	Hemostasis and thrombus formation.
	Angiogenic Regulators: IL8, Thrombospondin, Angiostatin, PF-4, TIMP-1,4, MMP-1,2,9, SDF-1, PMP Angiopoietin, Endostatin	Angiogenesis cascades and re-establishing vasculature.
	Cytokines: IL1, IL4, IL6, TFNα, SDF-1	Chemotaxis, inflammatory response modulation, and antimicrobial activity.
	Chemokines: RANTES, CXCL4, CXCL7, CCL2, CCL3, CCL5, β-TG	Inflammation, antimicrobial, and bactericidal activity.
	Complement Proteins: C3, C4	Phagocytosis, chemotaxis and platelet activation.
	Exosomes: mRNA, miRNA, CXCL4, CXCL7	Cell adhesion, paracrine communication, regulation of cell fate, and modulation of inflammatory response.
Dense granules	ADP, ATP, TFNα calcium, serotonin, epinephrine, pyrophosphates	Platelet activation and vasoconstriction.
Lysosomes	Collagenase, elastase, Cathepsin, α-arabinoside, β-galactosidase	Matrix degradation and antimicrobial activity.
Multivesicular Bodies	Exosomes Extracellular vesicles	Cell proliferation, PGF transportation, and platelet-cell communication.

Abbreviations: PDGF: platelet-derived growth factors; VEGF: vascular endothelial growth factor; TGF: transforming growth factor; FGF: fibroblast growth factor; EGF: epidermal growth factor; CTGF: connective tissue growth factor; vWF: von Willebrand factor; IL: interleukin; PF-4: platelet factor 4; TIMP: tissue inhibitor of metalloproteinase; MMP: matrix metalloproteinase; PMP: platelet-derived microparticles; TNF: tumor necrosis factor; SDF: stromal cell-derived factor; RANTES: regulated by T-Cell activation and probably secreted by T-Cells; CXCL: CXC chemokine ligand; CCL: C-C motif chemokine ligand; C: complement protein; ADP: adenosine diphosphate; ATP: adenosine triphosphate; mRNA: messenger RNA; miRNA: microRNA.

Adapted and modified from Everts, P.A.; Lana, J.F.; Alexander, R.W.; Dallo, I.; Kon, E.; Ambach, M.A.; van Zundert, A.; Podesta, L. Profound Properties of Protein-Rich, Platelet-Rich Plasma Matrices as Novel, Multi-Purpose Biological Platforms in Tissue Repair, Regeneration, and Wound Healing.

Leukocytes in PRP

The presence of leukocytes in PRP preparations depends on the processing device and preparation protocol. In plasma-based PRP devices, leukocytes are completely removed, while in buffy coat PRP preparations, they are significantly concentrated. Leukocytes play a critical role in the biology of acute and chronic tissue conditions due to their immune and host-defense mechanisms. The specific leukocyte composition in C-PRP can have significant cellular and tissue effects, as different PRP buffy coat systems produce varying ratios of neutrophils, lymphocytes, and monocytes. Eosinophils and basophils are not present in PRP formulations because their fragile cell membranes cannot withstand centrifugal processing forces.

Neutrophils

Neutrophils are vital leukocytes in healing pathways, creating barriers against pathogens in conjunction with antimicrobial proteins from platelets. Their presence in PRP depends on treatment objectives, as they can promote inflammation necessary for chronic wound care or bone healing. However, neutrophils can also have harmful effects, such as promoting fibrosis and weakening tendons by increasing the collagen type III to collagen type I ratio. Additionally, they release inflammatory cytokines and matrix metalloproteinases, which can have pro-inflammatory and catabolic effects on tissues.

Lymphocytes

Lymphocytes, particularly mononuclear T and B cells, are highly concentrated in C-PRP. They play a crucial role in cell-mediated cytotoxic adaptive immunity and can fight infections and adapt to intruders. T lymphocyte-derived cytokines (interferon-gamma and interleukin-4) strengthen macrophage polarization, indirectly contributing to tissue healing by modulating monocyte and macrophage differentiation.

Monocytes

Monocytes may be present or absent in PRP treatment vials, depending on the preparation device. They originate from bone marrow progenitor cells and can differentiate into macrophages or dendritic cells within the mononuclear phagocyte system. In degenerated tissues, monocytes differentiate into macrophages, which can have pro-inflammatory or pro-repair functions depending on the local environment. Monocyte-derived macrophages can switch between inflammatory (M1) and reparative (M2) phenotypes, with M2 macrophages promoting tissue repair and anti-inflammatory responses. PRP preparations rich in monocytes are likely to enhance tissue repair due to their immunomodulatory and cell-signaling capabilities.

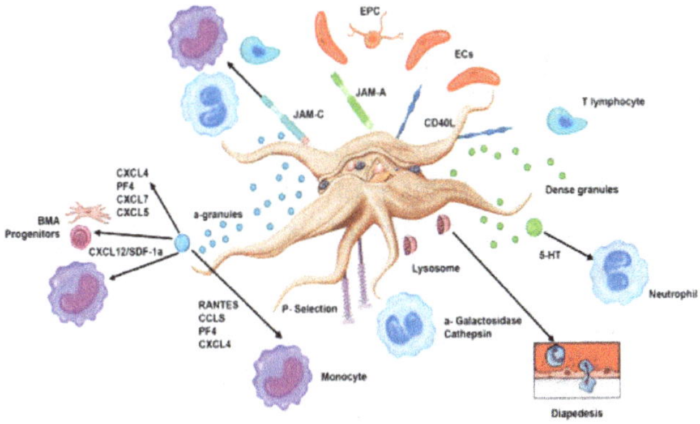

Figure 3.3 Activated PRP Platelet Pathways

Activated platelets stimulate cell proliferation; they contribute to chemotactic cell migration, incite immunomodulatory activities, contribute to angiogenesis, incite inflammatory activities, with the potential to stimulate the synthesis of mesenchymal and neurotrophic factors in order to stimulate tissue repair processes.

Abbreviations: BMA: bone marrow aspirate, EPC: endothelial progenitor cell, EC: endothelial cells, 5-HT: serotonin, RANTES: Regulated upon Activation Normal T Cell Expressed and Presumably Secreted, JAM: junctional adhesion molecules type, CD40L: cluster of differentiation 40 ligand, SDF-1: stromal cell-derived factor 1 alpha, CXCL: chemokine (C-X-C motif) ligand, PF4: platelet factor 4. Adapted and modified from Everts and colleagues (2020).

Platelet Adhesion Molecules

Platelet adhesion molecules play a critical role in the interaction of platelets with leukocytes, endothelial cells, and the extracellular matrix during immune responses. Integrins, like a5b1, LFA-2, and aIIbb3, are cell surface adhesion molecules that exist in a low-affinity state under normal conditions but transition to a high-affinity state upon activation. These integrins facilitate various interactions, such as the formation of platelet–leukocyte complexes, where integrin aIIbb3 binds to macrophage-1 antigen (Mac-1) on neutrophils via fibrinogen.

Additionally, the GP-Ib–V–IX complex on platelet membranes serves as the primary receptor for von Willebrand factor (vWF), mediating the initial contact of platelets with exposed subendothelial structures. Selectins, another class of adhesion molecules, are expressed on platelets (P-selectin) and neutrophils (L-selectin) under inflammatory conditions. P-selectin binds to its ligand PSGL-1 on neutrophils and monocytes, triggering intracellular signaling that activates neutrophil integrins Mac-1 and lymphocyte function-associated antigen-1 (LFA-1). This activation stabilizes neutrophil–platelet interactions, with Mac-1 binding to GPIb or GPIIb/IIIa on platelets via fibrinogen and LFA-1 binding to platelet intercellular adhesion molecule-2 for prolonged attachment.

PRP to Mimic the Onset of Healing

The term PRP was originally used in transfusion medicine to describe a platelet concentrate, where it remains in use today. Early clinical applications involved PRP as a fibrin tissue adhesive, with platelets valued mainly for enhancing fibrin polymerization and tissue sealing, rather than for stimulating healing. Over time, PRP preparations evolved to mimic the initiation of the natural healing cascade, gaining recognition for their capacity to deliver and release numerous growth factors, molecules, and other cytokines directly into the local tissue microenvironment. However, the potential role of PRP in delivering bioactive components and healing components is often overlooked. This situation was heightened by limited scientific evidence, commercial influences, overinflated claims, and the absence of standardized definitions or classifications. The biology of PRP is inherently complex, arguably more so than conventional pharmaceuticals. As living biomaterials, PRP preparations reflect the dynamic and adaptive nature of the patient's own blood, influenced by its cellular constituents and by the physiological state of the target tissue, whether acute or chronic. Consequently, clinical outcomes depend on both the intrinsic properties of the PRP and its interaction with the recipient's local microenvironment.

PRP Preparation Methods: Still Evolving

Multiple classification systems have been proposed to describe platelet-rich plasma (PRP) formulations, yet no universal framework exists for PRP or other autologous blood-derived products. An ideal classification would clearly define PRP characteristics, standardized terminology, and clinically relevant parameters to guide treatment selection for patient-specific conditions. In orthobiologics, PRP is commonly grouped into three categories: pure platelet-rich PRP (P-PRP), leukocyte-rich PRP (LR-PRP), and leukocyte-poor PRP (LP-PRP). While more specific than a generic "PRP" label, these categories lack detail regarding leukocyte composition—a critical factor in tissue biology and immune modulation. Specific leukocytes can influence tissue repair:

- Lymphocytes produce insulin-like growth factors and support remodeling.
- Monocytes and macrophages regulate inflammation

and promote repair.

- Neutrophils have uncertain roles, though some studies suggest they may enhance regeneration when combined with activated platelets.

Evidence on optimal formulations is mixed. For example, systematic reviews favor LP-PRP for osteoarthritis (OA), while others, such as Lana and colleagues, argue that certain leukocytes are beneficial for initiating regeneration via balanced pro- and anti-inflammatory signaling. PRP research is hindered by inconsistent reporting of preparation protocols, limiting reproducibility and comparison across studies. Many trials use "PRP" as a catch-all term, even for different formulations within the same indication. Progress has been made in understanding formulation variables—such as platelet dose, delivery routes, and cellular composition—but consensus on standardized PRP bioformulations remains essential for ensuring safe, targeted, and effective treatment.

Understanding *In Vitro* and *In Vivo* Platelet Dosing

The therapeutic potential of PRP and other platelet concentrate variations arises from the release of numerous growth factors, proteins, and bioactive molecules that drive tissue repair and regeneration. Upon activation, platelets form a temporary plug that serves as an extracellular matrix, supporting cell proliferation and differentiation. While it is reasonable to assume that higher platelet doses yield greater local concentrations of these factors, this relationship is not straightforward. Baseline platelet counts vary widely between patients, and preparation methods differ in how they concentrate and preserve platelets. Furthermore, some important PGFs, such as hepatocyte growth factor (HGF) and insulin-like growth factor 1 (IGF-1), are found in the plasma fraction, meaning their levels are unaffected by the PRP platelet dose.

In vitro studies have been widely used to explore platelet dosing because experimental parameters can be tightly controlled, and results obtained quickly. Many show a dose-dependent cellular response to PRP. However, Nguyen and Pham reported that excessively high growth factor concentrations may hinder, rather than enhance, cell activity. Other studies confirm that supraphysiological PGF levels can have detrimental effects, possibly due to a finite number of cell membrane receptors—once saturated, excess growth factors may disrupt normal cellular function.

The Significance of In Vitro Data on Platelet Concentrations

While *in vitro* studies offer valuable insights, they also have notable limitations. In living tissues, cell behavior is shaped by complex interactions between multiple cell types, three-dimensional architecture, and the surrounding extracellular matrix (ECM)—conditions that are difficult to replicate in two-dimensional monoculture systems. *In vitro* cell densities are often less than 1% of those found *in vivo*, altering signaling pathways. Standard culture techniques also fail to mimic physiological oxygen supply, homeostatic nutrient exchange, or waste clearance. As a result, laboratory conditions differ substantially from the *in vivo* environment, limiting the direct translation of PRP dosing data to clinical settings. Comparisons between *in vitro* findings and clinical results often reveal discrepancies. For example, Graziani and colleagues observed maximal osteoblast and fibroblast proliferation at platelet concentrations 2.5 times baseline *in vitro*, whereas Park and colleagues reported that a 5-fold increase was needed to achieve positive outcomes after spinal fusion. Similar inconsistencies have been noted between *in vitro* tendon cell proliferation studies and clinical outcome data, underscoring the challenges of extrapolating laboratory platelet concentration data to patient care.

Transitioning from Platelet Concentration to Platelet Dosing

The traditional focus on platelet concentration as a quality parameter for PRP has limitations, as it does not account for the total number of platelets delivered to the treatment site. Platelet dosing, which considers the platelet concentration multiplied by the injected PRP volume, provides a more accurate measure of the therapeutic dose. The DEPA classification defines dosing levels as very high (>5 billion platelets), high (3–5 billion platelets), medium (1–3 billion platelets), and low (<1 billion platelets). This approach allows for better correlation between platelet dose and patient outcomes, including tissue repair and angiogenesis.

PRP Device Variables and Considerations

The quality and efficacy of PRP injectates vary significantly due to differences in device design and preparation protocols, which affect the platelet and cellular yields. Some systems produce platelet concentrations lower than baseline whole blood levels, while dual-spin closed systems can achieve platelet concentrations exceeding $1.5 \times 10^6/\mu L$. Few PRP systems can deliver high platelet concentrations and allow for diverse bioformulations based on leukocyte and erythrocyte counts. To optimize PRP platelet dosing, factors such as the patient's baseline platelet concentration, pre-donated blood volume, and the PRP device platelet capture rate must be considered. Additionally, Oh and colleagues found that dual-spin methods produce higher platelet concentrations and greater levels of VEGF and PDGF compared to single-spin methods, due to their superior platelet capture rates.

Gravitational Cellular Density Separation and Platelet Dose

Dual-spin PRP devices use gravitational cellular density separation to concentrate blood cells based on size and density, producing a buffy-coat layer rich in platelets and other cellular components. This method contrasts with single-spin devices, which yield an acellular plasma layer lacking leukocytes and erythrocytes. The platelet capture rate, PRP volume, and preparation volume are critical factors in achieving optimal platelet dosing. Several studies have shown that the PRP platelet dose is important in determining patient outcomes. Low platelet dosages can negatively impact angiogenesis and tissue repair, while higher platelet doses have been shown to stimulate cell-cell interactions and support tissue repair processes in a dose-dependent manner.

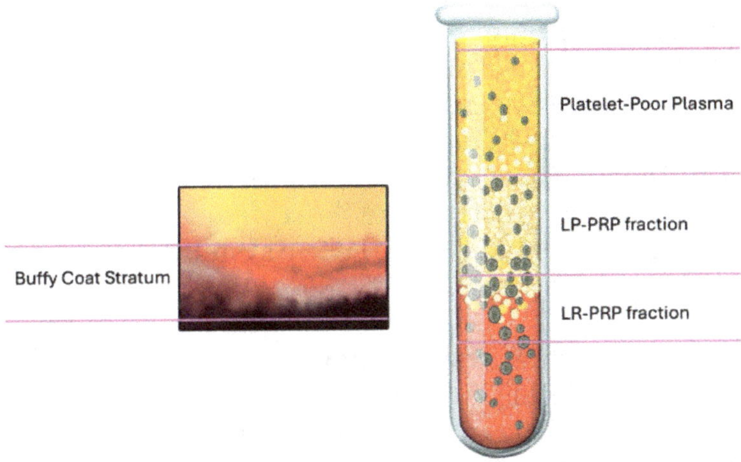

Simplified graphic of whole blood density separation,
With magnification of a buffy coat stratum in a PRP preparation.

Figure 3.4 Buffy Coat Stratum after Whole Blood Centrifugation Density Separation

This illustration demonstrates the density-based separation of whole blood following centrifugation during PRP preparation. The upper layer consists primarily of platelet-poor plasma (PPP), while the platelet-rich plasma fractions are concentrated closer to the buffy coat. The magnified image highlights the buffy coat stratum, a transitional layer enriched with platelets and varying concentrations of leukocytes located between the plasma and red blood cell layers. Depending on the preparation technique and collection method, clinicians may selectively harvest leukocyte-poor PRP (LP-PRP) or leukocyte-rich PRP (LR-PRP) for therapeutic applications.

Platelets and Leukocytes Play Pivotal Roles in Innate and Adaptive Immune Responses

Platelets and leukocytes are essential for initiating and regulating immune responses in both innate and adaptive immunity. The body's ability to detect foreign bodies and injured tissues triggers the wound healing cascade and inflammatory pathways. In the innate immune system, monocytes, macrophages, neutrophils, and natural killer cells play critical roles, while lymphocytes and their subsets are central to the adaptive immune system. These immune cells work together to protect the host from infection, with overlapping functions between the two systems.

Innate Immune System

The innate immune system plays a critical role in non-specifically identifying invading microbes or tissue damage and initiating their clearance. This process is triggered when pattern recognition receptors (PRRs), such as Toll-like receptors (TLRs), bind to pathogen-associated molecular patterns (PAMPs) or damage-associated molecular patterns (DAMPs). Activation of PRRs stimulates the transcription factor nuclear factor kappa B (NF-kappa-B), which regulates immune responses in both innate and adaptive immunity. Platelets also contribute to this system by expressing immunomodulatory receptors, including P-selectin, CD40 ligand (CD40L), cytokines (e.g., IL-1beta, TGF-beta), and platelet-specific TLRs, enabling interactions with immune cells.

Platelets are among the first responders to endothelial injury and microbial invasion, aggregating and releasing platelet agonists like ADP, thrombin, and vWF. This activation promotes the expression of chemokine receptors, facilitating rapid platelet accumulation at infection or injury sites. Neutrophils, monocytes, and dendritic cells (DCs) are key innate immune cells recruited during this process. Platelet-leukocyte interactions regulate inflammation, wound healing, and tissue repair, particularly in regenerative medicine applications using platelet-rich plasma (PRP). TLR-4 on platelets stimulates platelet-neutrophil interactions, modulating the release of reactive oxygen species (ROS) and myeloperoxidase (MPO) during the leukocyte oxidative burst. Platelet-neutrophil interactions also lead to neutrophil degranulation and the formation of neutrophil extracellular traps (NETs), which trap and kill bacteria through NETosis. Monocytes, upon activation, migrate to damaged tissues, secreting inflammatory molecules that influence chemotaxis and proteolytic activity. Platelets further enhance monocyte function by inducing NF-kappa-B activation and promoting the oxidative burst, facilitated by CD40L-MAC-1 interactions. Additionally, platelet-derived chemokines like PF4, RANTES, IL-1beta, and CXCL-12 prevent monocyte apoptosis and drive their differentiation into macrophages. Dendritic cells, derived from bone marrow precursors, bridge the innate and adaptive immune systems. They recognize pathogens and tissue damage, migrate to secondary lymphoid organs, and present antigens to activate T lymphocytes. Platelets recruit DCs through interactions involving immunoglobulin JAM receptors and MAC-1 integrins 96. Following exposure to platelet-derived growth factors, DCs differentiate, playing a vital role in immune response amplification.

Adaptive Immune System

The adaptive immune system, which is specific and antigen-driven, takes over after the innate immune system identifies microbes or tissue damage. This system involves B lymphocytes (B cells) that bind antigens and regulatory T lymphocytes (Tregs) that coordinate pathogen elimination. T cells are categorized into helper T cells (Th cells) and cytotoxic T cells (Tc cells). Th cells include Th1, Th2, and Th17 subtypes, which secrete pro-inflammatory cytokines such as IFN-gamma, TNF-beta, and interleukins (e.g., IL-17). These cells are critical in combating intracellular infections and stimulating the proliferation and differentiation of immune cells involved in the response. Tc cells, on the other hand, eliminate targeted microbes and cells. Th2 cells produce IL-4, which promotes M2 macrophage polarization toward a regenerative phenotype, while IFN-gamma shifts macrophages toward the inflammatory M1 phenotype, depending on cytokine dose and timing. IL-4 activation of M2 macrophages induces Treg cells to differentiate into Th2 cells, creating a positive feedback loop that enhances IL-4 production. Th cells also guide macrophages toward pro-regenerative phenotypes in response to tissue-derived biologics, playing a significant role in controlling inflammation and tissue repair.

Platelets contribute to adaptive immunity by facilitating interactions with leukocytes, promoting monocyte and macrophage responses, and supporting the maturation of dendritic cells (DCs) and natural killer (NK) cells, which in turn activate specific T- and B-cell responses. Platelet granular components, including CD40L, are critical for modulating adaptive immunity by aiding antigen presentation and influencing T-cell responses. Platelets regulate CD4 T cell responses in a complex manner, promoting both pro- and anti-inflammatory responses to inflammatory stimuli. Platelets enhance T cell-dependent B-cell responses by linking T-cell and B-cell interactions via CD40-CD40L. Additionally, platelets express numerous surface receptors that, upon activation, release inflammatory and bioactive molecules from their granules, influencing both innate and adaptive immune responses.

A Role for Platelet-Derived Serotonin in PRP and Painkilling

Platelet-derived serotonin (5-hydroxytryptamine, 5-HT) plays a significant role in PRP, with critical functions in both the central and peripheral systems. While serotonin is well-known for its role in the central nervous system (CNS), particularly in pain regulation, the majority of the body's serotonin is produced in the gastrointestinal tract and circulated in the bloodstream, where it is stored in platelet dense granules at high concentrations (65 mmol/L). Peripheral serotonin regulates various biological functions in multiple organ systems, including cardiovascular, pulmonary, gastrointestinal, genitourinary, and platelet function. It also acts as an immune modulator, influencing inflammation and immune cells through specific serotonin receptors (5HTRs). Serotonin exerts its effects through interaction with 5HTRs, a superfamily comprising seven members (5-HT1 to 7) and at least fourteen receptor subtypes. During platelet degranulation, activated platelets release serotonin, which promotes vasoconstriction and stimulates the activation of neighboring platelets and lymphocytes via 5HTRs expressed on endothelial, smooth muscle, and immune cells. Serotonin has mitogenic effects on vascular endothelial cells, potentially supporting angiogenesis and tissue repair by stimulating the growth of damaged blood vessels. The autocrine effects of platelet-derived serotonin enhance platelet activation and recruit circulating platelets, initiating signaling cascades that support platelet reactivity. In the immune system, serotonin functions as an immunomodulator, regulating both innate and adaptive immune responses through its interaction with various leukocytes. Depending on the 5HTRs expressed on immune cells, platelet-derived serotonin can stimulate Treg proliferation, regulate B cell function, and influence the activity of natural killer cells and neutrophils. It also recruits dendritic cells (DCs) and monocytes to inflammatory sites. The use of concentrated PRP, with platelet concentrations exceeding 1 × 106/μL, could deliver high levels of platelet-derived serotonin to inflammatory sites, potentially modulating immune cell functions and influencing clinical outcomes in inflammatory conditions.

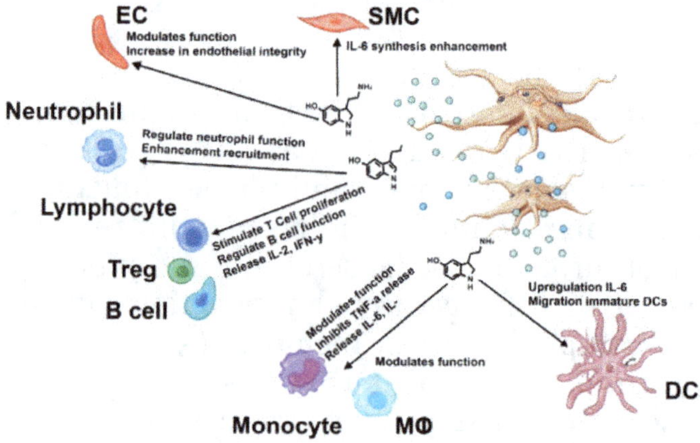

Figure 3.5 The Central Functional Role of 5-HT in PRP Platelets

The complex 5-HT-mediated effects following inflammatory platelet activation are multifaceted. Upon activation, platelets release their granular contents, including 5-HT from dense granules. This 5-HT release triggers a cascade of diverse responses affecting immune, endothelial, and smooth muscle cells.

Abbreviations: SMC: smooth muscle cell, EC: endothelial cell, Treg: regular T lymphocyte, MF: macrophage, DC: dendritic cell, IL: interleukin, IFN-y: interferon gamma.

Analgesic effects

PRP has demonstrated significant analgesic effects, attributed to the release of various pro- and anti-inflammatory mediators from activated platelets. These mediators can both induce and reduce pain, depending on the context. PRP alters the microenvironment at the site of application, influencing tissue repair and regeneration through complex pathways involving anabolic and catabolic processes, cell proliferation, differentiation, and stem cell regulation. These characteristics have made PRP a promising treatment for chronic pain conditions such as sports injuries, orthopedic pathologies, spinal disorders, and chronic wounds, although the exact mechanisms remain not fully understood. In 2008, Everts and colleagues conducted a randomized controlled trial on the analgesic effects of PRP in shoulder surgery. They observed a significant reduction in pain scores, decreased opioid use, and improved post-surgical rehabilitation. The study highlighted the role of platelet-released serotonin (5-HT) in pain modulation. Activated platelets release 5-HT from dense granules, which can modulate pain through various serotonin receptors (5-HT1, 5-HT2, 5-HT3, 5-HT4, and 5-HT7) in peripheral tissues. This release of 5-HT from PRP, particularly in concentrated formulations like PRP, is believed to contribute to its analgesic effects. Endogenous 5-HT, released from platelets, mast cells, and endothelial cells in response to tissue injury or trauma, plays a critical role in nociceptive transmission. The 5-HT system can both increase and decrease pain intensity following noxious stimulation, with central and peripheral regulation of nociceptive signals influenced by alterations in the 5-HT system. This has led to the development of drugs like selective serotonin reuptake inhibitors (SSRIs), which inhibit serotonin reuptake and affect the duration and intensity of serotonin signaling, offering an alternative treatment for chronic pain. Clinical and animal studies on PRP's analgesic effects have shown mixed results. Some studies report little to no pain relief in conditions like tendinosis or rotator cuff tears, while others indicate significant pain reduction in tendinosis, osteoarthritis (OA), plantar fasciitis, and other foot and ankle disorders. The effectiveness of PRP in pain relief is influenced by factors such as platelet concentration, biocellular composition, delivery methods, activation protocols, and the type of tissue treated. Notably, these studies by Kuffler and others have shown that PRP can promote axonal regeneration and target reinnervation, leading to long-term pain relief in patients with chronic neuropathic pain. In these cases, pain reduction was observed within weeks after PRP application and persisted for years. Additionally, PRP has shown analgesic effects in post-surgical wound care and skincare, with studies demonstrating reduced pain and enhanced angiogenesis in PRP-treated patients compared to controls.

Despite promising results, the optimal PRP platelet concentration for maximal pain relief is still unknown. Animal studies suggest that higher platelet concentrations may lead to more effective pain relief, but further clinical research is needed to determine the ideal PRP formulation and its mechanisms of action in chronic and degenerative pain conditions.

Angiogenesis Effects Following PRP Application

PRP preparations in orthobiological and regenerative medicine therapies facilitate the delivery of various biomolecules released by platelets and other cells, such as leukocytes, to target tissue sites. This process initiates cascades that promote immunomodulation, inflammation, and angiogenesis, all of which are essential for tissue healing and repair.

Angiogenesis is a dynamic, multi-step process involving the formation and organization of new microvessels from existing blood vessels. It relies on several biological mechanisms, including endothelial cell migration, proliferation, differentiation, and division. These processes are crucial for the growth of new blood vessels, which restore blood flow and support the high metabolic demands of tissue repair and regeneration by delivering oxygen and nutrients while removing waste products.

Pro- and Anti-Angiogenic PRP Platelet Properties

Angiogenic activities are regulated by pro-angiogenic factors like vascular endothelial growth factor (VEGF) and anti-angiogenic factors such as thrombospondin-1 (TSP-1). TSP-1, present in PRP at concentrations of approximately 183.3 ± 21.6 μg/mL, can inhibit endothelial cell proliferation at higher concentrations (>15%).

In diseased microenvironments, platelet-rich plasma (PRP) can restore angiogenic balance. PRP contains multiple growth factors, including VEGF, basic-FGF, and TGF-β, which stimulate endothelial cell tubulogenesis and new blood vessel formation. TSP-1, also present in PRP, plays a dual role by activating latent TGF-β and modulating VEGF signaling. Studies have shown that PRP constituents increase Tie2 phosphorylation in mouse lungs, accelerating compensatory lung growth after pneumonectomy. The angiogenic potential of PRP may contribute to healing in poorly vascularized musculoskeletal tissues, such as menisci and tendons.

Angiogenesis Following PRP is Dose-dependent

PRP therapies have gained recognition for their angiogenic effects, crucial in tissue repair and regeneration. PRP delivers concentrated PGFs and cytokines that stimulate angiogenesis, vasculogenesis, and arteriogenesis. Studies have shown that PRP enhances endothelial cell proliferation, migration, and tube formation, while the optimal platelet concentration for promoting angiogenesis was identified as 1.5×10^6 platelets/μL *in vitro*. However, excessive platelet concentrations may inhibit angiogenesis, emphasizing the importance of precise platelet dosing.

PRP's angiogenic effects are concentration-dependent, with low concentrations (<5%) promoting cell proliferation. The angiogenic balance is further regulated by factors like TGF-β, which can have both pro- and anti-angiogenic effects. PRP has been shown to stimulate endothelial cell proliferation, migration, and tube formation *in vitro* and promote angiogenesis *in vivo*, highlighting its potential in therapeutic angiogenesis for various conditions in tissue repair and regeneration.

Key mechanisms include:

1. SDF-1a binds to CXCR4 receptors on endothelial progenitor cells, enhancing neovascularization.

2. VEGF stimulation of endothelial cell proliferation and capillary formation.

3. Synergy between multiple PGFs (e.g., PDGF-BB and VEGF) accelerates mature vascular network formation.

Conclusion

Technological advancements in PRP devices and preparation methods have shown promising results in patient outcomes, although there is still a lack of clarity regarding different PRP bioformulations and their biological properties. The full potential of PRP applications and indications remains to be determined.

This chapter emphasizes the need for standardization and classification in PRP preparation methods to achieve some level of consensus regarding the optimization of PRP bioformulations and, therefore, more consistent patient outcomes. However, there is increasing agreement on the optimal platelet dosing concentrations needed to support functional tissue repair. The chapter also explores the role of PGFs and the mechanisms of action of platelets, including their interactions with leukocytes, and the consequences for the immune system, painkilling effects, and angiogenesis. The contributing therapeutic effects of the various leukocytes and their synergetic effects in PRP preparations are still poorly understood and remain controversial. Some studies suggest LR-PRP may increase inflammatory responses compared to LP-PRP. However, leukocytes may also contribute beneficial effects through interactions with platelets and the release of regulatory factors. The precise mechanisms and synergistic effects of different leukocyte populations in PRP are not fully understood and require further well-designed clinical studies to fully understand the therapeutic potential of PRP across various applications.

Bibliography

Acosta-Rodriguez, E. V., Napolitani, G., Lanzavecchia, A., & Sallusto, F. (2007). Interleukins 1β and 6 but not transforming growth factor-β are essential for the differentiation of interleukin 17–producing human T helper cells. *Nature Immunology*, *8*(9), 942–949. https://doi.org/10.1038/ni1496

Alberts, B. (Ed.). (2002). *Molecular biology of the cell* (4th ed.). Garland Science.

Amable, P., Carias, R. B., Teixeira, M. V., da Cruz Pacheco, Í., Corrêa do Amaral, R. J., Granjeiro, J., & Borojevic, R. (2013). Platelet-rich plasma preparation for regenerative medicine: Optimization and quantification of cytokines and growth factors. *Stem Cell Research & Therapy*, *4*(3), Article 67. https://doi.org/10.1186/scrt218

Andia, I., & Maffulli, N. (2018). A contemporary view of platelet-rich plasma therapies: Moving toward refined clinical protocols and precise indications. *Regenerative Medicine*, *13*(6), 717–728. https://doi.org/10.2217/rme-2018-0042

Arreola, R., Becerril-Villanueva, E., Cruz-Fuentes, C., Velasco-Velázquez, M. A., Garcés-Alvarez, E. M., Hurtado-Alvarado, G., Quintero-Fabian, S., & Pavón, L. (2015). Immunomodulatory effects mediated by serotonin. *Journal of Immunology Research*, *2015*, Article 354957. https://doi.org/10.1155/2015/354957

Balagholi, S., Rezaei Kanavi, M., Alizadeh, S., Dabbaghi, R.,

Karami, S., Kheiri, B., & Ahmadieh, H. (2018). Effects of fibrin glue as a three-dimensional scaffold in cultivated adult human retinal pigment epithelial cells. *Journal of Biomaterials Applications*, *33*(4), 514–526. https://doi.org/10.1177/0885328218799793

Banu, S. A., & Sharun, K. (2025). Minimum reporting requirements for platelet-rich plasma in biomaterial research. *Biomaterials Advances*, *175*, Article 214314. https://doi.org/10.1016/j.bioadv.2025.214314

Bennett, J. S. (2005). Structure and function of the platelet integrin αIIbβ3. *The Journal of Clinical Investigation*, *115*(12), 3363–3369. https://doi.org/10.1172/JCI26989

Berger, M., Gray, J. A., & Roth, B. L. (2009). The expanded biology of serotonin. *Annual Review of Medicine*, *60*(1), 355–366. https://doi.org/10.1146/annurev.med.60.042307.110802

Berndt, S., Carpentier, G., Turzi, A., Borlat, F., Cuendet, M., & Modarressi, A. (2021). Angiogenesis is differentially modulated by platelet-derived products. *Biomedicines*, *9*(3), Article 251. https://doi.org/10.3390/biomedicines9030251

Bir, S. C., Esaki, J., Marui, A., Sakaguchi, H., Kevil, C. G., Ikeda, T., Komeda, M., & Sakata, R. (2011). Therapeutic treatment with sustained-release platelet-rich plasma restores blood perfusion by augmenting ischemia-induced angiogenesis and arteriogenesis in diabetic mice. *Journal of Vascular Research*, *48*(3), 195–205. https://doi.org/10.1159/000318793

Blair, P., & Flaumenhaft, R. (2009). Platelet α-granules: Basic biology and clinical correlates. *Blood Reviews*, *23*(4), 177–189. https://doi.org/10.1016/j.blre.2009.04.001

Chahla, J., Cinque, M. E., Piuzzi, N. S., Mannava, S., Geeslin, A. G., Murray, I. R., & Laprade, R. F. (2017). A call for standardization in platelet-rich plasma preparation protocols and composition reporting: A systematic review of the clinical orthopaedic literature. *The Journal of Bone and Joint Surgery*, *99*(20), 1769–1779. https://doi.org/10.2106/JBJS.16.01374

Clark, S. R., Ma, A. C., Tavener, S. A., McDonald, B., Goodarzi, Z., Kelly, M. M., Patel, K. D., Chakrabarti, S., McAvoy, E., Sinclair, G. D., Keys, E. M., Allen-Vercoe, E., DeVinney, R., Doig, C. J., Green, F. H. Y., & Kubes, P. (2007). Platelet TLR4 activates neutrophil extracellular traps to ensnare bacteria in septic blood. *Nature Medicine*, *13*(4), 463–469. https://doi.org/10.1038/nm1565

Clemetson, K. J., Clemetson, J. M., Proudfoot, A. E. I., Power, C. A., Baggiolini, M., & Wells, T. N. C. (2000). Functional expression of CCR1, CCR3, CCR4, and CXCR4 chemokine receptors on human platelets. *Blood*, *96*(13), 4046–4054. https://doi.org/10.1182/blood.V96.13.4046

Cognasse, F., Laradi, S., Berthelot, P., Bourlet, T., Marotte, H., Mismetti, P., Garraud, O., & Hamzeh-Cognasse, H. (2019). Platelet inflammatory response to stress. *Frontiers in Immunology*, *10*, Article 1478. https://doi.org/10.3389/fimmu.2019.01478

Collins, T., Alexander, D., & Barkatali, B. (2021). Platelet-rich plasma: A narrative review. *EFORT Open Reviews*, *6*(4), 225–235. https://doi.org/10.1530/EOR-20-0017

Dale, D. C., Boxer, L., & Liles, W. C. (2008). The phagocytes: Neutrophils and monocytes. *Blood*, *112*(4), 935–945. https://doi.org/10.1182/blood-2007-12-077917

Das, A., Sinha, M., Datta, S., Abas, M., Chaffee, S., Sen, C. K., & Roy, S. (2015). Monocyte and macrophage plasticity in tissue repair and regeneration. *The American Journal of Pathology*, *185*(10), 2596–2606. https://doi.org/10.1016/j.ajpath.2015.06.012

de Melo, B. A. G., Luzo, Â. C. M., Lana, J. F. S. D., & Santana, M. H. A. (2019). Centrifugation conditions in the L-PRP preparation affect soluble factors release and mesenchymal stem cell proliferation in fibrin nanofibers. *Molecules*, *24*(15), Article 2729. https://doi.org/10.3390/molecules24152729

de Mos, M. (2009). *Tendon cell behavior and matrix remodeling in degenerative tendinopathy* [Doctoral dissertation, Erasmus University Rotterdam]. s.n.

Deppermann, C., & Kubes, P. (2018). Start a fire, kill the bug: The role of platelets in inflammation and infection.

Innate Immunity, *24*(6), 335–348. https://doi.org/10.1177/1753425918789255

Diacovo, T. G., deFougerolles, A. R., Bainton, D. F., & Springer, T. A. (1994). A functional integrin ligand on the surface of platelets: Intercellular adhesion molecule-2. *The Journal of Clinical Investigation*, *94*(3), 1243–1251. https://doi.org/10.1172/JCI117442

Duerschmied, D., Suidan, G. L., Demers, M., Herr, N., Carbo, C., Brill, A., Cifuni, S. M., Kollussery, M., Wagner, D. D., & Fuchs, T. A. (2013). Platelet serotonin promotes the recruitment of neutrophils to sites of acute inflammation in mice. *Blood*, *121*(6), 1008–1015. https://doi.org/10.1182/blood-2012-06-437392

Dutzmann, J., Korte, T., & Langer, H. F. (2018). The platelet response to tissue injury. *Frontiers in Medicine*, *5*, Article 317. https://doi.org/10.3389/fmed.2018.00317

Etulain, J., Mena, H. A., Meiss, R. P., Frechtel, G., Gutt, S., Negrotto, S., & Schattner, M. (2018). An optimised protocol for platelet-rich plasma preparation to improve its angiogenic and regenerative properties. *Scientific Reports*, *8*(1), Article 1513. https://doi.org/10.1038/s41598-018-19912-3

Everts, P., Onishi, K., Jayaram, P., Lana, J. F., & Mautner, K. (2020). Platelet-rich plasma: New performance understandings and therapeutic considerations in 2020 [Preprint]. *Preprints*. https://doi.org/10.20944/preprints202010.0069.v1

Everts, P. A., Devilee, R. J. J., Brown Mahoney, C., van Erp, A., Oosterbos, C. J. M., Stellenboom, M., Knape, J. T. A., & van Zundert, A. (2008). Exogenous application of platelet-leukocyte gel during open subacromial decompression contributes to improved patient outcome. *European Surgical Research, 40*(2), 203–210. https://doi.org/10.1159/000110862

Everts, P. A., Flanagan, G., & Podesta, L. (2022). Autologous orthobiologics. In S. A. Mostoufi, T. K. George, & A. J. Tria (Eds.), *Clinical guide to musculoskeletal medicine* (pp. 651–679). Springer International Publishing. https://doi.org/10.1007/978-3-030-92042-5_62

Everts, P. A., Hoffmann, J., Weibrich, G., Mahoney, C. B., Schönberger, J. P. A. M., van Zundert, A., & Knape, J. T. A. (2006). Differences in platelet growth factor release and leucocyte kinetics during autologous platelet gel formation. *Transfusion Medicine, 16*(5), 363–368. https://doi.org/10.1111/j.1365-3148.2006.00692.x

Everts, P. A., Lana, J. F., Alexander, R. W., Dallo, I., Kon, E., Ambach, M. A., Buford, D., Peng, J., Mahmood, A., & Podesta, L. (2024). Profound properties of protein-rich, platelet-rich plasma matrices as novel, multi-purpose biological platforms in tissue repair, regeneration, and wound healing. *International Journal of Molecular Sciences, 25*(14), Article 7914. https://doi.org/10.3390/ijms25147914

Everts, P. A., Lana, J. F., Onishi, K., Buford, D., Peng, J.,

Mahmood, A., Dallo, I., Podesta, L., & Alexander, R. W. (2023). Angiogenesis and tissue repair depend on platelet dosing and bioformulation strategies following orthobiological platelet-rich plasma procedures: A narrative review. *Biomedicines, 11*(7), Article 1922. https://doi.org/10.3390/biomedicines11071922

Everts, P. A., Mazzola, T., Mautner, K., Randelli, P. S., & Podesta, L. (2022). Modifying orthobiological PRP therapies are imperative for the advancement of treatment outcomes in musculoskeletal pathologies. *Biomedicines, 10*(11), Article 2933. https://doi.org/10.3390/biomedicines10112933

Everts, P. A., Podesta, L., & Alexander, R. W. (2024). A comprehensive guide of cellular blood-derived and mesenchymal stem cell-based autologous biological preparations for tissue repair, regeneration, and wound healing. In P. A. Everts & R. W. Alexander (Eds.), *Pearls in biological and molecular tissue repair pathways*. IntechOpen. https://doi.org/10.5772/intechopen.1177070

Everts, P. A. M., Knape, J. T. A., Weibrich, G., Hoffmann, J., Overdevest, E. P., Box, H. A. M., & van Zundert, A. (2006). Platelet-rich plasma and platelet gel: A review. *The Journal of Extra-Corporeal Technology, 38*(2), 174–187.

Fadadu, P. P., Mazzola, A. J., Hunter, C. W., & Davis, T. T. (2019). Review of concentration yields in commercially available platelet-rich plasma (PRP) systems: A call for PRP standardization. *Regional Anesthesia & Pain Medicine*, *44*(6), 652–659. https://doi.org/10.1136/rapm-2018-100356

Fedorova, N. V., Ksenofontov, A. L., Serebryakova, M. V., Stadnichuk, V. I., Gaponova, T. V., Baratova, L. A., & Sud'ina, G. F. (2018). Neutrophils release metalloproteinases during adhesion in the presence of insulin, but cathepsin G in the presence of glucagon. *Mediators of Inflammation*, *2018*, Article 5917410. https://doi.org/10.1155/2018/5917410

Ferrante, C. J., & Leibovich, S. J. (2012). Regulation of macrophage polarization and wound healing. *Advances in Wound Care*, *1*(1), 10–16. https://doi.org/10.1089/wound.2011.0307

Freire-Garabal, M., Núñez, M. J., Balboa, J., López-Delgado, P., Gallego, R., García-Caballero, T., Fernández-Roel, R., & Mayán, J. M. (2003). Serotonin upregulates the activity of phagocytosis through 5-HT1A receptors. *British Journal of Pharmacology*, *139*(2), 457–463. https://doi.org/10.1038/sj.bjp.0705273

Gaudino, S. J., & Kumar, P. (2019). Cross-talk between antigen presenting cells and T cells impacts intestinal homeostasis, bacterial infections, and tumorigenesis. *Frontiers in Immunology*, *10*, Article 360. https://doi.org/10.3389/fimmu.2019.00360

Gentile, P., Calabrese, C., De Angelis, B., Pizzicannella, J.,

Kothari, A., & Garcovich, S. (2019). Impact of the different preparation methods to obtain human adipose-derived stromal vascular fraction cells (AD-SVFs) and human adipose-derived mesenchymal stem cells (AD-MSCs): Enzymatic digestion versus mechanical centrifugation. *International Journal of Molecular Sciences, 20*(21), Article 5471. https://doi.org/10.3390/ijms20215471

Gentile, P., & Garcovich, S. (2020). Systematic review—The potential implications of different platelet-rich plasma (PRP) concentrations in regenerative medicine for tissue repair. *International Journal of Molecular Sciences, 21*(16), Article 5702. https://doi.org/10.3390/ijms21165702

Giusti, I., D'Ascenzo, S., Mancò, A., Di Stefano, G., Di Francesco, M., Rughetti, A., Pavan, A., & Dolo, V. (2014). Platelet concentration in platelet-rich plasma affects tenocyte behavior in vitro. *BioMed Research International, 2014*, Article 630870. https://doi.org/10.1155/2014/630870

Giusti, I., Rughetti, A., D'Ascenzo, S., Millimaggi, D., Pavan, A., Dell'Orso, L., & Dolo, V. (2009). Identification of an optimal concentration of platelet gel for promoting angiogenesis in human endothelial cells. *Transfusion, 49*(4), 771–778. https://doi.org/10.1111/j.1537-2995.2008.02033.x

Graziani, F., Ivanovski, S., Cei, S., Ducci, F., Tonetti, M., &

Gabriele, M. (2006). The in vitro effect of different PRP concentrations on osteoblasts and fibroblasts. *Clinical Oral Implants Research*, *17*(2), 212–219. https://doi.org/10.1111/j.1600-0501.2005.01203.x

Guillibert, C., Charpin, C., Raffray, M., Benmenni, A., Dehaut, F. X., El Ghobeira, G., ... & Magalon, J. (2019). Single injection of high volume of autologous pure PRP provides a significant improvement in knee osteoarthritis: A prospective routine care study. *International Journal of Molecular Sciences*, *20*(6), Article 1327. https://doi.org/10.3390/ijms20061327

Hara, G. R., & Basu, T. (2014). Platelet-rich plasma in regenerative medicine. *Journal of Spine*, *3*, Article 185. https://doi.org/10.22074/CELLJ.2023.558213.1093

Hsu, C. W., Yuan, K., & Tseng, C. C. (2009). The negative effect of platelet-rich plasma on the growth of human cells is associated with secreted thrombospondin-1. *Oral Surgery, Oral Medicine, Oral Pathology, Oral Radiology, and Endodontology*, *107*(2), 185–192. https://doi.org/10.1016/j.tripleo.2008.08.019

Iberg, C. A., & Hawiger, D. (2020). Natural and induced tolerogenic dendritic cells. *The Journal of Immunology*, *204*(4), 733–744. https://doi.org/10.4049/jimmunol.1901002

Kaiko, G. E., Horvat, J. C., Beagley, K. W., & Hansbro, P. M. (2008). Immunological decision-making: How does the immune system decide to mount a helper T-cell response? *Immunology*, *123*(3), 326–338. https://doi.org/10.1111/j.1365-2567.2007.02719.x

Kakudo, N., Morimoto, N., Kushida, S., Ogawa, T., & Kusumoto, K. (2014). Platelet-rich plasma releasate promotes angiogenesis in vitro and in vivo. *Medical Molecular Morphology*, *47*(2), 83–89. https://doi.org/10.1007/s00795-013-0038-x

Kellouche, S., Mourah, S., Bonnefoy, A., Schoëvaert, D., Podgorniak, M. P., Calvo, F., Dosquet, C., & Legrand, C. (2007). Platelets, thrombospondin-1 and human dermal fibroblasts cooperate for stimulation of endothelial cell tubulogenesis through VEGF and PAI-1 regulation. *Experimental Cell Research*, *313*(4), 786–799. https://doi.org/10.1016/j.yexcr.2006.11.011

Kim, J. H., Park, Y. B., Ha, C. W., Roh, Y. J., & Park, J. G. (2021). Adverse reactions and clinical outcomes for leukocyte-poor versus leukocyte-rich platelet-rich plasma in knee osteoarthritis: A systematic review and meta-analysis. *Orthopaedic Journal of Sports Medicine*, *9*(6), Article 23259671211011307. https://doi.org/10.1177/23259671211011307

Kingsley, C. S. (1954). Blood coagulation; evidence of an antagonist to factor VI in platelet-rich human plasma. *Nature*, *173*(4407), 723–724. https://doi.org/10.1038/173723a0

Kobayashi, Y., Saita, Y., Nishio, H., Ikeda, H., Takazawa, Y., Nagao, M., Kaneko, K., & Ning, L. (2016). Leukocyte concentration and composition in platelet-rich plasma (PRP) influences the growth factor and protease concentrations. *Journal of Orthopaedic Science, 21*(5), 683–689. https://doi.org/10.1016/j.jos.2016.07.009

Kuffler, D. P. (2015). Platelet-rich plasma promotes axon regeneration, wound healing, and pain reduction: Fact or fiction. *Molecular Neurobiology, 52*(2), 990–1014. https://doi.org/10.1007/s12035-015-9251-x

Kuffler, D. P. (2019). Variables affecting the potential efficacy of PRP in providing chronic pain relief. *Journal of Pain Research, 12*, 109–116. https://doi.org/10.2147/JPR.S190065

Kurita, J., Miyamoto, M., Ishii, Y., Aoyama, J., Takagi, G., Naito, Z., ... & Mizuno, K. (2011). Enhanced vascularization by controlled release of platelet-rich plasma impregnated in biodegradable gelatin hydrogel. *The Annals of Thoracic Surgery, 92*(6), 2180–2187. https://doi.org/10.1016/j.athoracsur.2011.07.027

Lana, J. F. (2019). Leukocyte-rich PRP versus leukocyte-poor PRP - The role of monocyte/macrophage function in the healing cascade. *Journal of Clinical Orthopaedics and Trauma, 10*(Suppl 1), S6. https://doi.org/10.1016/j.jcot.2019.05.008

Lana, J. F., Purita, J., Everts, P. A., De Mendonça Neto, P. A. T., De Moraes Ferreira Jorge, D., Mosaner, T., ... & Santana, M. H. A. (2023). Platelet-rich plasma power-mix gel (PPM)—An orthobiologic optimization protocol rich in growth factors and fibrin. *Gels*, *9*(7), Article 553. https://doi.org/10.3390/gels9070553

Lana, J. F. S. D., Purita, J., Paulus, C., Huber, S. C., Rodrigues, B. L., Rodrigues, A. A., ... & Belangero, W. D. (2017). Contributions for classification of platelet rich plasma – proposal of a new classification: MARSPILL. *Regenerative Medicine*, *12*(5), 565–574. https://doi.org/10.2217/rme-2017-0045

Lit, K. K., Zhirenova, Z., & Blocki, A. (2024). Insulin-like growth factor-binding protein 7 (IGFBP7): A microenvironment-dependent regulator of angiogenesis and vascular remodeling. *Frontiers in Cell and Developmental Biology*, *12*, Article 1421438. https://doi.org/10.3389/fcell.2024.1421438

Lin, M. T., Wei, K. C., & Wu, C. H. (2020). Effectiveness of platelet-rich plasma injection in rotator cuff tendinopathy: A systematic review and meta-analysis of randomized controlled trials. *Diagnostics*, *10*(4), Article 189. https://doi.org/10.3390/diagnostics10040189

Lutz, C., Cheng, J., Prysak, M., Zukofsky, T., Rothman, R., & Lutz, G. (2022). Clinical outcomes following intradiscal injections of higher-concentration platelet-rich plasma in patients with chronic lumbar discogenic pain. *International Orthopaedics*, *46*(6), 1381–1388. https://doi.org/10.1007/s00264-022-05389-y

Magalon, J., Brandin, T., Francois, P., Degioanni, C., De Maria,

L., Grimaud, F., ... & Sabatier, F. (2021). Technical and biological review of authorized medical devices for platelets-rich plasma preparation in the field of regenerative medicine. *Platelets*, *32*(2), 200–208. https://doi.org/10.1080/09537104.2020.1732101

Magalon, J., Chateau, A. L., Bertrand, B., Louis, M. L., Silvestre, A., Giraudo, L., ... & Sabatier, F. (2016). DEPA classification: A proposal for standardising PRP use and a retrospective application of available devices. *BMJ Open Sport & Exercise Medicine*, *2*(1), Article e000060. https://doi.org/10.1136/bmjsem-2015-000060

Mammadova-Bach, E., Mauler, M., Braun, A., & Duerschmied, D. (2018). Autocrine and paracrine regulatory functions of platelet serotonin. *Platelets*, *29*(6), 541–548. https://doi.org/10.1080/09537104.2018.1478458

Marrazzo, P., Paduano, F., Palmieri, F., Marrelli, M., & Tatullo, M. (2016). Highly efficient in vitro reparative behaviour of dental pulp stem cells cultured with standardised platelet lysate supplementation. *Stem Cells International*, *2016*, Article 7230140. https://doi.org/10.1155/2016/7230140

Mohammadi, S., Nasiri, S., Mohammadi, M. H., Malek Mohammadi, A., Nikbakht, M., Zahed Panah, M., & Atashi, A. (2017). Evaluation of platelet-rich plasma gel potential in acceleration of wound healing duration in patients underwent pilonidal sinus surgery: A randomized controlled parallel clinical trial.

Transfusion and Apheresis Science, 56(2), 226–232. https://doi.org/10.1016/j.transci.2016.12.001

Moojen, D. J. F., Schure, R. M., Overdevest, E. P., van Zundert, A., Knape, J. T. A., Castelein, R. M., ... & Dhert, W. J. A. (2008). Antimicrobial activity of platelet-leukocyte gel against *Staphylococcus aureus*. *Journal of Orthopaedic Research, 26*(3), 404–410. https://doi.org/10.1002/jor.20519

Newton, K., & Dixit, V. M. (2012). Signaling in innate immunity and inflammation. *Cold Spring Harbor Perspectives in Biology, 4*(3), Article a006049. https://doi.org/10.1101/cshperspect.a006049

Nguyen, P. A., & Pham, T. A. V. (2018). Effects of platelet-rich plasma on human gingival fibroblast proliferation and migration in vitro. *Journal of Applied Oral Science, 26*, Article e20180048. https://doi.org/10.1590/1678-7757-2018-0048

Ojea-Pérez, A. M., Acebes-Huerta, A., Arias-Fernández, T., Gutiérrez, L., & Muñoz-Turrillas, M. C. (2019). Implementation of a closed platelet-rich-plasma preparation method using the local blood bank infrastructure at the Principality of Asturias (Spain): Back to basic methodology and a demographics perspective after 1 year. *Transfusion and Apheresis Science, 58*(5), 650–655. https://doi.org/10.1016/j.transci.2019.08.016

Odem, M. A., Bavencoffe, A. G., Cassidy, R. M., Lopez, E. R.,

Tian, J., Dessauer, C. W., ... & Walters, E. T. (2018). Isolated nociceptors reveal multiple specializations for generating irregular ongoing activity associated with ongoing pain. *Pain, 159*(11), 2347–2362. https://doi.org/10.1097/j.pain.0000000000001341

Ogle, M. E., Segar, C. E., Sridhar, S., & Botchwey, E. A. (2016). Monocytes and macrophages in tissue repair: Implications for immunoregenerative biomaterial design. *Experimental Biology and Medicine, 241*(10), 1084–1097. https://doi.org/10.1177/1535370216650293

Oh, J. H., Kim, W., Park, K. U., & Roh, Y. H. (2015). Comparison of the cellular composition and cytokine-release kinetics of various platelet-rich plasma preparations. *The American Journal of Sports Medicine, 43*(12), 3062–3070. https://doi.org/10.1177/0363546515607773

Pakala, R., Willerson, J. T., & Benedict, C. R. (1994). Mitogenic effect of serotonin on vascular endothelial cells. *Circulation, 90*(4), 1919–1926. https://doi.org/10.1161/01.CIR.90.4.1919

Papait, A., Cancedda, R., Mastrogiacomo, M., & Poggi, A. (2018). Allogeneic platelet-rich plasma affects monocyte differentiation to dendritic cells causing an anti-inflammatory microenvironment, putatively fostering wound healing. *Journal of Tissue Engineering and Regenerative Medicine, 12*(1), e515–e526.

https://doi.org/10.1002/term.2319

Park, M. S., Moon, S. H., Kim, T. H., Oh, J. K., Yoon, W. Y., & Chang, H. G. (2018). Platelet-rich plasma for the spinal fusion. *Journal of Orthopaedic Surgery*, *26*(1), Article 2309499018755771. https://doi.org/10.1177/2309499018755771

Patetsos, E., & Horjales-Araujo, E. (2016). Treating chronic pain with SSRIs: What do we know? *Pain Research and Management*, *2016*, Article 2020915. https://doi.org/10.1155/2016/2020915

Petraglia, F., Florio, P., Nappi, C., & Genazzani, A. R. (1996). Peptide signaling in human placenta and membranes: Autocrine, paracrine, and endocrine mechanisms. *Endocrine Reviews*, *17*(2), 156–186. https://doi.org/10.1210/edrv-17-2-156

Piao, L., Park, H., & Jo, C. H. (2017). Theoretical prediction and validation of cell recovery rates in preparing platelet-rich plasma through a centrifugation. *PLOS ONE*, *12*(11), Article e0187509. https://doi.org/10.1371/journal.pone.0187509

Richardson, T. P., Peters, M. C., Ennett, A. B., & Mooney, D. J. (2001). Polymeric system for dual growth factor delivery. *Nature Biotechnology*, *19*(11), 1029–1034. https://doi.org/10.1038/nbt1101-1029

Rosenthal, N. E., Mazzanti, C. M., Barnett, R. L., Hardin, T. A., Turner, E. H., Lam, G. K., ... & Goldman, D. (1998). Role of serotonin transporter promoter repeat length polymorphism (5-HTTLPR) in seasonality and seasonal affective disorder. *Molecular Psychiatry*, *3*(2), 175–177. https://doi.org/10.1038/sj.mp.4000366

Rossaint, J., & Zarbock, A. (2015). Platelets in leucocyte recruitment and function. *Cardiovascular Research*, *107*(3), 386–395. https://doi.org/10.1093/cvr/cvv102

Rossi, L. A., Murray, I. R., Chu, C. R., Muschler, G. F., Rodeo, S. A., & Piuzzi, N. S. (2019). Classification systems for platelet-rich plasma. *The Bone & Joint Journal*, *101-B*(8), 891–896. https://doi.org/10.1302/0301-620X.101B8.BJJ-2019-0037.R1

Ruggeri, Z. M., & Mendolicchio, G. L. (2007). Adhesion mechanisms in platelet function. *Circulation Research*, *100*(12), 1673–1685. https://doi.org/10.1161/01.RES.0000267878.97021.b1

Sadtler, K., Estrellas, K., Allen, B. W., Wolf, M. T., Fan, H., Tam, A. J., ... & Elisseeff, J. H. (2016). Developing a pro-regenerative biomaterial scaffold microenvironment requires T helper 2 cells. *Science*, *352*(6283), 366–370. https://doi.org/10.1126/science.aad5672

Samadi, P., Sheykhhasan, M., & Khoshinani, H. M. (2019). The use of platelet-rich plasma in aesthetic and regenerative medicine: A comprehensive review. *Aesthetic Plastic Surgery*, *43*(3), 803–814. https://doi.org/10.1007/s00266-019-01393-y

Sansores-España, L. D., Melgar-Rodríguez, S., Vernal, R.,

Carrillo-Ávila, B. A., Martínez-Aguilar, V. M., & Díaz-Zúñiga, J. (2022). Neutrophil N1 and N2 subsets and their possible association with periodontitis: A scoping review. *International Journal of Molecular Sciences, 23*(20), Article 12068. https://doi.org/10.3390/ijms232012068

Scheuerer, B., Ernst, M., Dürrbaum-Landmann, I., Fleischer, J., Grage-Griebenow, E., Brandt, E., ... & Flad, H. D. (2000). The CXC-chemokine platelet factor 4 promotes monocyte survival and induces monocyte differentiation into macrophages. *Blood*, *95*(4), 1158–1166. https://doi.org/10.1182/blood.V95.4.1158.004k37_1158_1166

Semple, J. W., Italiano, J. E., & Freedman, J. (2011). Platelets and the immune continuum. *Nature Reviews Immunology*, *11*(4), 264–274. https://doi.org/10.1038/nri2956

Silverberg, G. D., Harbury, C. B., & Rubenstein, E. (1977). A physiological sealant for cerebrospinal fluid leaks. *Journal of Neurosurgery*, *46*(2), 215–219. https://doi.org/10.3171/jns.1977.46.2.0215

Smadja, D. M., d'Audigier, C., Bièche, I., Evrard, S., Mauge, L., Dias, J. V., ... & Gaussem, P. (2011). Thrombospondin-1 is a plasmatic marker of peripheral arterial disease that modulates endothelial progenitor cell angiogenic properties. *Arteriosclerosis, Thrombosis, and Vascular*

Biology, *31*(3), 551–559. https://doi.org/10.1161/ATVBAHA.110.220624

Tang, Y. Q., Yeaman, M. R., & Selsted, M. E. (2002). Antimicrobial peptides from human platelets. *Infection and Immunity*, *70*(12), 6524–6533. https://doi.org/10.1128/IAI.70.12.6524-6533.2002

The GRIP (Groupe de Recherche sur les Injections de PRP)., Eymard, F., Ornetti, P., Maillet, J., Noel, É., Adam, P., ... & Richette, P. (2020). Intra-articular injections of platelet-rich plasma in symptomatic knee osteoarthritis: A consensus statement from French-speaking experts. *Knee Surgery, Sports Traumatology, Arthroscopy*, *28*(10), 3183–3192. https://doi.org/10.1007/s00167-020-06102-5

Ubezio, G., & Ghio, M. (2014). Bio-modulators in platelet-rich plasma: A comparison of the amounts in products from healthy donors and patients produced with three different techniques. *Blood Transfusion*, *12*(Suppl 1), s319–s321. https://doi.org/10.2450/2012.0128-12

Vahabi, S., Yadegari, Z., & Mohammad-Rahimi, H. (2017). Comparison of the effect of activated or non-activated PRP in various concentrations on osteoblast and fibroblast cell line proliferation. *Cell and Tissue Banking*, *18*(3), 347–353. https://doi.org/10.1007/s10561-017-9640-4

Van Gils, J. M., Zwaginga, J. J., & Hordijk, P. L. (2009). Molecular and functional interactions among monocytes, platelets, and endothelial cells and their relevance for cardiovascular diseases. *Journal of Leukocyte Biology*, *85*(2), 195–204. https://doi.org/10.1189/jlb.0708401

Vasina, E. M., Cauwenberghs, S., Feijge, M. A. H., Heemskerk, J. W. M., Weber, C., & Koenen, R. R. (2011). Microparticles from apoptotic platelets promote resident macrophage differentiation. *Cell Death & Disease*, *2*(9), Article e211. https://doi.org/10.1038/cddis.2011.94

Wan, M., Ding, L., Wang, D., Han, J., & Gao, P. (2020). Serotonin: A potent immune cell modulator in autoimmune diseases. *Frontiers in Immunology*, *11*, Article 186. https://doi.org/10.3389/fimmu.2020.00186

Weirather, J., Hofmann, U. D. W., Beyersdorf, N., Ramos, G. C., Vogel, B., Frey, A., ... & Frantz, S. (2014). Foxp3+ CD4+ T cells improve healing after myocardial infarction by modulating monocyte/macrophage differentiation. *Circulation Research*, *115*(1), 55–67. https://doi.org/10.1161/CIRCRESAHA.115.303895

Woodell-May, J. E., & Sommerfeld, S. D. (2020). Role of inflammation and the immune system in the progression of osteoarthritis. *Journal of Orthopaedic Research*, *38*(2), 253–257. https://doi.org/10.1002/jor.24457

Wu, W. P., Hao, J. X., Xu, X. J., Wiesenfeld-Hallin, Z., Koek,

W., & Colpaert, F. C. (2003). The very-high-efficacy 5-HT1A receptor agonist, F 13640, preempts the development of allodynia-like behaviors in rats with spinal cord injury. *European Journal of Pharmacology*, *478*(2–3), 131–137. https://doi.org/10.1016/j.ejphar.2003.08.070

Wynn, T. A., & Vannella, K. M. (2016). Macrophages in tissue repair, regeneration, and fibrosis. *Immunity*, *44*(3), 450–462. https://doi.org/10.1016/j.immuni.2016.02.015

Xiong, Y., Gong, C., Peng, X., Liu, X., Su, X., Tao, X., ... & Hu, Y. (2023). Efficacy and safety of platelet-rich plasma injections for the treatment of osteoarthritis: A systematic review and meta-analysis of randomized controlled trials. *Frontiers in Medicine, 10*, Article 1204144. https://doi.org/10.3389/fmed.2023.1204144

Yoshida, M., Funasaki, H., & Marumo, K. (2016). Efficacy of autologous leukocyte-reduced platelet-rich plasma therapy for patellar tendinopathy in a rat treadmill model. *Muscles, Ligaments and Tendons Journal*, *6*(2), 205–215.

Younas, M., Hue, S., Lacabaratz, C., Guguin, A., Wiedemann, A., Surenaud, M., ... & Lelievre, J. D. (2013). IL-7 modulates in vitro and in vivo human memory T regulatory cell functions through the CD39/ATP axis. *The Journal of Immunology*, *191*(6), 3161–3168.

https://doi.org/10.4049/jimmunol.1301015

Yuan, T., Zhang, C. Q., & Wang, H. C. (2013). Augmenting tendon and ligament repair with platelet-rich plasma (PRP). *Muscles, Ligaments and Tendons Journal*, *3*(3), 139–144. https://doi.org/10.11138/mltj/2013.3.3.139

Zirlik, A., Maier, C., Gerdes, N., MacFarlane, L., Soosairajah, J., Bavendiek, U., ... & Schönbeck, U. (2007). CD40 ligand mediates inflammation independently of CD40 by interaction with Mac-1. *Circulation*, *115*(12), 1571–1580. https://doi.org/10.1161/CIRCULATIONAHA.106.683318

CHAPTER 4

The PRP Treatment Process—What to Expect

Authors: Robert Engelen

Orthobiologics is a form of regenerative medicine that uses natural substances from your own body to help reduce pain and support healing. One of the most commonly used orthobiologic treatments is **Platelet-Rich Plasma (PRP)**.

PRP is created from your own blood and is designed to stimulate your body's natural repair process. If you have decided to move forward with PRP, this chapter will guide you through **exactly what to expect**—from scheduling your appointment, to the day of the procedure, and through the recovery period afterwards.

Knowing what is coming helps reduce anxiety and allows you to feel confident and actively involved in your care.

What to Expect Before the Procedure

Initial Evaluation: Setting the Foundation

Your PRP journey starts with a thorough evaluation by your

provider. This visit is one of the most important steps in the process.

During your appointment, your provider will:

- Review your medical history
- Discuss previous injuries, surgeries, and treatments
- Review medications and supplements you are taking
- Perform a physical exam focused on the painful area

Imaging studies such **as X-rays, ultrasound, or MRI scans** may be reviewed or ordered if needed. These images help confirm the diagnosis and allow your provider to target the PRP injection accurately.

You will also discuss your goals. Whether your goal is to reduce chronic pain, improve movement, return to activity, or delay surgery, clearly defining expectations helps customize the treatment plan specifically for you.

Pre-Injection Instructions: Optimizing Your Platelets

PRP works best when your platelets are healthy and active. Certain medications and supplements can interfere with platelet function, so preparation is important.

In the days leading up to your procedure:

- **Stop anti-inflammatory medications (NSAIDs)** such as ibuprofen (Advil), naproxen (Aleve), and aspirin **5–7 days before your procedure**, unless otherwise directed
- If you take **daily aspirin for heart or vascular conditions**, speak with your prescribing doctor before stopping

- **Extra Strength Tylenol is allowed** for pain relief (do not exceed 3,000 mg in 24 hours, but always check with your treating provider)
- On the day of the procedure, **650 mg of Tylenol may be taken one hour before**, if advised
- Avoid **corticosteroid injections** at the treatment site for at least **1–2 months prior**
- Avoid **oral or systemic steroids** for at least **1 month prior**
- Avoid these supplements for **1 week prior**:
    - Vitamin E
    - Fish oil or flax oil
    - Vitamin A
    - Turmeric or curcumin
    - Aloe
    - Garlic
    - Astaxanthin
- Avoid **smoking and alcohol** for one week before the procedure
- **Hydrate well**:
    - At least four 8-oz glasses of water the day before
    - At least four 8-oz glasses within three hours of your appointment
- If you take **blood thinners** such as **Eliquis, Xarelto, Pradaxa**, or similar medications, your provider will communicate with your primary care doctor or cardiologist. In some cases, it may not be safe to stop

these medications. For **high thrombotic risk** (recent stents, AFib, mechanical valves), consult cardiology—it may not be safe to hold. Please use a **shared decision-making** approach with your treating physician.

These steps help ensure your PRP is as effective as possible.

What to Wear and Bring

On the day of your procedure:

- Wear **loose, comfortable clothing** that allows easy access to the treatment area
    - A tank top or loose shirt for shoulder treatments
- Arrange for **transportation home**, especially if numbing medication or relaxation medication is used
- Bring a friend or family member if helpful for support

Blood Draw Preparation: Maximizing PRP Quality

Because PRP comes from your own blood, hydration and circulation matter.

To optimize platelet quality:

- Aim for **64 ounces of water** the day of your appointment (unless advised otherwise)
- Some patients may benefit from **light or brief high-intensity exercise** earlier in the day—discuss this with your provider first

Pre-Procedure Patient Checklist

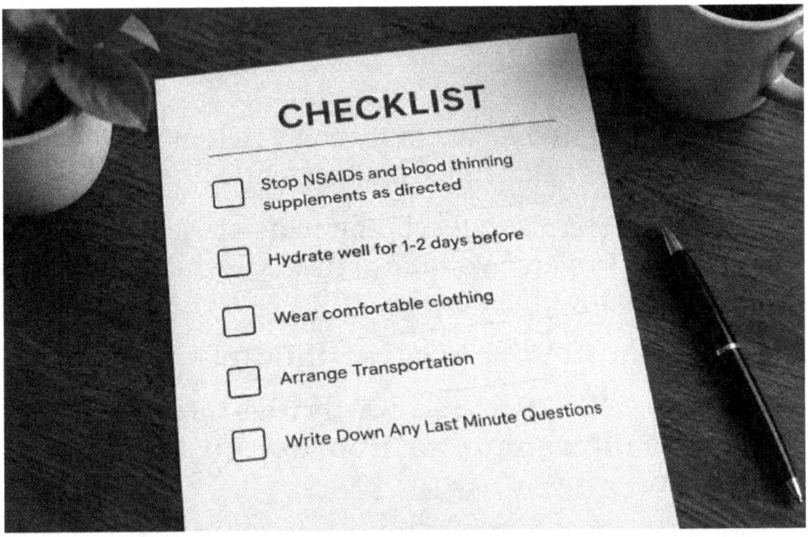

Figure 4.1 Patient Preparation Checklist Prior to PRP Treatment

This checklist highlights common pre-procedure recommendations for patients preparing to undergo PRP therapy, including discontinuation of certain medications and supplements as directed, adequate hydration, appropriate attire, transportation planning, and preparation of questions for discussion with the treating physician. Proper preparation may help optimize the treatment experience and facilitate procedural efficiency.

How PRP Injections Are Performed

Step-by-Step: What Happens During the Procedure

The PRP procedure begins with a simple blood draw, similar to what you would experience during routine lab work. The blood is then placed into a centrifuge, a machine that spins rapidly to separate the blood into layers. Your provider may do a single or double spin in the centrifuge.

These layers include:

- Red blood cells (RBCs)
- Plasma
- A concentrated layer (buffy coat) rich in platelets (and white blood cells, called leukocytes)

Your provider carefully collects the platelet-rich portion and suspends it in a targeted volume of plasma, which is then used immediately for the injection.

Image Guidance: Why Accuracy Matters

To ensure the PRP is delivered exactly where it is needed, your provider uses **ultrasound or fluoroscopy (real-time X-ray)** guidance.

This allows the provider to:

- See the injured tissue in real time
- Avoid nearby nerves or blood vessels
- Place PRP precisely into the joint, tendon, or ligament

Accurate placement is one of the most important factors in treatment success.

Injection Technique Overview

Before the injection:

- The skin is cleaned thoroughly with an antiseptic solution
- Local numbing medication may be used to improve comfort

The injection itself usually takes **only a few minutes**. PRP can be injected into joints, tendons, ligaments, or other targeted structures, depending on your condition.

Sterility and Safety

PRP is considered a **low-risk procedure**, especially when performed by trained providers.

Safety measures include:

- Sterile technique
- Single-use or sterilized equipment
- Image guidance for accuracy

Because PRP comes from your own blood, allergic reactions are extremely rare.

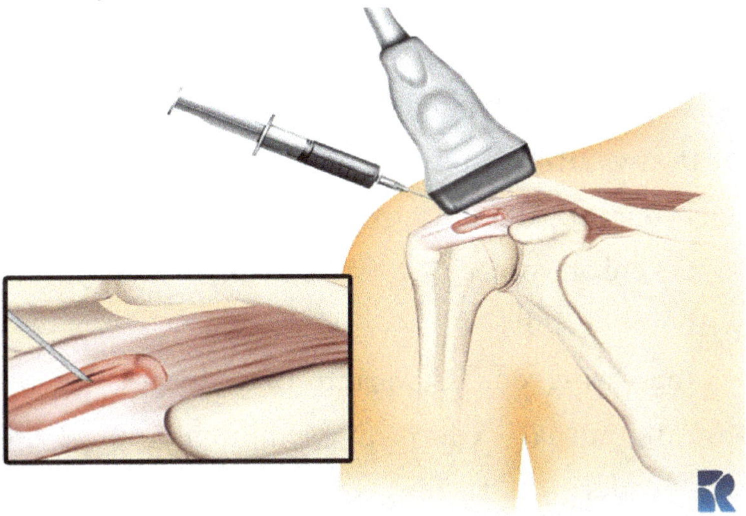

Figure 4.2 Ultrasound-Guided PRP Treatment for a Partial Rotator Cuff Tear

This illustration demonstrates an ultrasound-guided PRP injection targeting a partial-thickness tear of the supraspinatus tendon at its insertion on the greater tuberosity. Ultrasound guidance allows real-time visualization of the tendon pathology and precise needle placement into the region of degeneration or tearing, facilitating accurate delivery of the biologic injectate while minimizing injury to surrounding structures.

What Happens After PRP?

Expected Sensations: What's Normal

After your injection, it is normal to experience:

- Soreness or stiffness
- A feeling of pressure or fullness
- Temporary increase in pain ("flare response") for 1–3 days

This flare is expected and is a sign that your body's healing response has been activated.

Red Flags vs. Reassurance

Contact your provider if you experience:

- Severe or worsening pain lasting more than 72 hours
- Fever or chills
- Increasing redness, warmth, or drainage
- Any unusual or concerning symptoms

Your provider will review what is normal and when to call—never hesitate to reach out.

The First 24–48 Hours: Take It Easy

During the first couple of days:

- Avoid strenuous or high-impact activity
- Gentle movement is usually encouraged
- Avoid NSAIDs unless instructed otherwise

- Icing is generally discouraged
- Heat with a heating pad for comfort is encouraged

Inflammation plays a role in healing, and PRP relies on this natural process.

Immediate Post-Procedure Recommendations

Home Care Tips

To support healing response:

- Stay well hydrated
- Eat an **anti-inflammatory diet** with whole foods and vegetables
- Prioritize good sleep

When to Start Moving Again

Depending on the treated area, gentle stretching or range-of-motion exercises may begin **immediately**. Physical therapy is often introduced in a **phased and controlled manner**.

Your provider will guide you on:

- When to start therapy
- What movements to avoid
- How to progress safely

Proper rehabilitation significantly improves PRP outcomes.

Post-PRP Care Checklist

✓ Stay hydrated
✓ Avoid NSAIDs
✓ Eat anti-inflammatory foods
✓ Rest, but don't completely immobilize
✓ Follow your rehab plan

Preparing Yourself: Confidence and Expectations

Common Patient Questions

"Will it hurt?"

Some discomfort is expected, but numbing options are available.

"When will I feel better?"

Improvement often begins within a few weeks, with continued progress over months.

"What if it doesn't work?"

PRP can be repeated and combined with other treatments if needed. It is one part of a comprehensive care plan.

Mental Preparation and Healing Mindset

Healing takes time. PRP is not an instant fix, but a process. Progress may come in small steps—less pain, better movement, improved sleep.

Staying patient, engaged, and optimistic plays an important role in recovery. Trust the process and communicate openly with your care team.

PRP Frequently Asked Questions (Extended Patient FAQs)

How is PRP different from stem cell therapy?

PRP uses **platelets from your own blood**, which contain growth factors that help modulate inflammation and support healing. Stem cell treatments use different cells and are typically more invasive and costly. PRP is often a first-line regenerative option before considering more advanced therapies.

Will PRP cure my condition?

PRP is not a cure-all. Its goal is to **reduce pain, improve function, and support healing**. Many patients experience meaningful improvement, but results vary based on the condition, severity, and overall health.

Can PRP be repeated?

Yes. PRP can safely be repeated if needed. Some patients benefit from a **series of injections**, while others improve after just one. Speaking with your provider about the latest literature, along with the condition being treated, will help to drive decision-making.

Can I go back to work after PRP?

Many patients return to desk or light-duty work the same or the next day. Jobs involving heavy lifting or repetitive motion may require temporary restrictions.

Can PRP make things worse?

Temporary soreness or a flare response is common and expected. Serious complications are rare when PRP is performed correctly and with image guidance.

Does age matter with PRP?

PRP can be effective at many ages. While younger patients may heal faster, older patients often still benefit—especially when PRP is used to modulate inflammation and slow degeneration.

Do I need imaging before PRP?

Yes. Imaging, such as ultrasound, X-ray, or MRI, helps confirm the diagnosis and ensures PRP is placed in the correct structure.

Why is ultrasound guidance important?

Accurate placement improves results. Anatomic or 'blind'

injections can miss the target, reducing effectiveness. Ultrasound allows real-time visualization for precision.

Is PRP experimental?

PRP has been used for decades in orthopedics, sports medicine, dentistry, and surgery. While it is not yet standardized across all specialties, the body of research supporting PRP continues to grow.

PRP Recovery Timeline: What to Expect

PRP healing happens in **phases**, not overnight. Understanding the timeline helps set realistic expectations.

Day 0–3: The Inflammatory Phase

- Injection-site soreness
- Temporary increase in pain ("flare")
- Mild stiffness or swelling
- Rest and gentle ROM movement only

✓ This phase is **expected and necessary** for healing

Week 1–2: Early Phase

- Pain begins to settle
- Improved comfort with daily activities
- Gentle range-of-motion exercises may begin
- No NSAIDs (consider discontinuing NSAID use for 4–6 weeks)

✓ Many patients begin noticing early improvement

Weeks 3–6: Tissue Repair Phase

- Continued pain reduction

- Improved strength and mobility
- Physical therapy often progresses
- Increased activity tolerance

✓ Tissue Healing is activated beneath the surface

Weeks 6–12: Remodeling Phase

- Tendons and joints become stronger
- Functional improvements become more noticeable
- Return to sport or higher-level activity may begin (guided)

✓ This is where **long-term benefits** are built

3–6 Months: Maximal Benefit

- Peak improvement for most patients
- Ongoing strengthening and conditioning
- Possible repeat PRP if needed

✓ Improvement continues even when pain is gone

Bibliography

Barile, A., La Marra, A., Arrigoni, F., Mariani, S., & Zugaro, L. (2016). Anaesthetics, steroids and platelet-rich plasma (PRP) in ultrasound-guided musculoskeletal procedures. *British Journal of Radiology, 89*(1065), Article 20150344. https://doi.org/10.1259/bjr.20150344

Chalidis, B., Givissis, P., Papadopoulos, P., & Pitsilos, C. (2023). Molecular and biologic effects of platelet-rich plasma (PRP) in ligament and tendon healing and regeneration: A systematic review. *International Journal of Molecular Sciences, 24*(3), Article 2744. https://doi.org/10.3390/ijms24032744

Charlesworth, J., Fitzpatrick, J., Perera, N. K. P., & Orchard, J. (2019). Osteoarthritis — a systematic review of long-term safety implications for osteoarthritis of the knee. *BMC Musculoskeletal Disorders, 20*, Article 151. https://doi.org/10.1186/s12891-019-2525-0

Cherian, C., Malanga, G. A., & Mautner, K. (2020). Optimizing platelet-rich plasma (PRP) injections: A narrative review. *Biologic Orthopedics Journal, 2*(1), e14.

Everts, P. A., Onishi, K., Jayaram, P., Lana, J. F., & Mautner, K. (2020). Platelet-rich plasma: New performance understandings and therapeutic considerations in 2020. *International Journal of Molecular Sciences, 21*(20), Article 7794. https://doi.org/10.3390/ijms21207794

Grémeaux, V., Lamontagne, M., Bélanger, V., Dalmais, E., & Noël, É. (2026). Rehabilitation and return to activity after platelet-rich plasma injections in chronic tendinopathies: Consensus from international experts. *PM&R*. Advance online publication. https://doi.org/10.1002/pmrj.13111

Hsu, W. K., Mishra, A., Rodeo, S., Fu, F. H., & Terry, M. A. (2013). Platelet-rich plasma in orthopaedic applications: Evidence-based recommendations for treatment. *Journal of the American Academy of Orthopaedic Surgeons*, *21*(12), 739–748. https://doi.org/10.5435/JAAOS-21-12-739

Marques, L. F., Stessuk, T., Camargo, I. C. C., Sabeh, N., & dos Santos, L. (2015). Platelet-rich plasma (PRP): Methodological aspects and clinical applications. *Platelets*, *26*(2), 101–113. https://doi.org/10.3109/09537104.2014.881991

Mautner, K., Malanga, G. A., & Colberg, R. E. (2011). Optimization of ingredients, procedures and rehabilitation for platelet-rich plasma injections for chronic tendinopathy. *Pain Management*, *1*(6), 523–532.

Sampson, S., Gerhardt, M. B., & Mandelbaum, B. (2008). Platelet rich plasma injection grafts for musculoskeletal injuries: A review. *Current Reviews in Musculoskeletal Medicine*, *1*(3–4), 165–174. https://doi.org/10.1007/s12178-008-9032-5

CHAPTER 5

Scientific Literature for PRP & Common Shoulder Conditions

Authors: Steve Schaaf, Sarah Allen & Michael Greenberg

PRP for Rotator Cuff Injuries: Clinical Studies

Overview of Key Studies

Rotator cuff disorders are the most common cause of shoulder pain and dysfunction, with a higher prevalence in those who participate in repetitive overhead motions, along with the aging process. There are several different subtypes of rotator cuff injuries, with the most common being tendinopathies and tears. Tendinopathies can either involve inflammation of the tendon, known as tendinitis, or degeneration of the tendon, known as tendinosis. In comparison to tendinopathies, tears involve disruption of the tendon fibers, which can range from partial to complete tears. It is important to differentiate these types of rotator cuff injuries, as treatment options and prognosis can vary.

Several clinical studies and reviews have examined how PRP helps with rotator cuff injuries, including tendinopathies and tears:

- A study of 150 patients with rotator cuff tendinopathies found that those who received leukocyte-rich PRP injections experienced improved shoulder scores, including pain measured by the VAS pain scale and function measured by the ASES. Similar improvements were seen in daily activity performance and satisfaction with the treatment. In addition, none of the patients' rotator cuff pathology worsened after treatment.
- A meta-analysis of 552 patients with rotator cuff tendinopathy showed that PRP injections led to significantly lower pain scores and better shoulder function than treatments like dry needling or physical therapy alone. This review included both leukocyte-rich (LR-PRP) and leukocyte-poor (LP-PRP) formulations, suggesting benefits across multiple PRP types.
- Another study with 30 patients who underwent ultrasound-guided PRP injections versus corticosteroid injections for rotator cuff tendinopathy showed more meaningful improvements in pain and function shortly after treatment in those who received a PRP injection.
- For people with partial rotator cuff tears, a systematic review of randomized controlled trials involving 516 patients showed an improvement in pain and overall shoulder function regardless of PRP injection site, including intra-articular, subacromial, or intratendinous.
- Another systematic review and meta-analysis of 641 patients with partial rotator cuff tears looked at PRP in the setting of non-operative treatment and found that

people receiving PRP had significantly better shoulder function than those who did not undergo this treatment.

- A two-year study in which 71 patients with rotator cuff tendinopathies received PRP injections exceeded the Minimal Clinically Important Difference in pain and Quick Disabilities of Arm, Shoulder & Hand (Q-DASH) scores.
- An additional meta-analysis involving 923 patients who underwent a surgical repair of their torn rotator cuff showed that the use of adjunct PRP led to:

  Significantly fewer retears

  Statistically better Constant-Murley scores

  Statistically better UCLA scores

  Greater improvement in VAS pain scores

Improvements in Pain, Strength, and Function

Across studies, PRP has been shown to help reduce pain and improve shoulder function, including mobility and strength. Researchers often use the following outcome tools:

- VAS (Visual Analog Scale): Patients reported less shoulder pain after PRP injections.
- ASES (American Shoulder and Elbow Surgeons) score: This score improved in most PRP-treated groups, indicating better function in daily activities.
- Constant-Murley Score: While not in every study, when used, this measure also improved, reflecting gains in strength and range of motion.
- Improved muscle integrity in previously injured rotator cuff tendons.

These findings suggest that PRP can help patients return to regular activities with less discomfort and better shoulder function.

Optimal Protocols from the Literature

Researchers are still working to determine the best way to prepare and deliver PRP, but what has emerged from the literature so far is:

- Dosing and Frequency: Most studies used 1–2 injections, spaced a few weeks apart. Some improvements were seen as early as a few weeks after the first injection.
- Injection Volume: The volume injected varied slightly (often between 2 and 5 mL), depending on the injury, including the size of the tendon tear being treated.
- Leukocyte Content: Some studies used leukocyte-rich PRP (LR-PRP) while others used leukocyte-poor PRP (LP-PRP). Early evidence suggests that LP-PRP may reduce inflammation more effectively and lead to better outcomes in rotator cuff healing.
- Injection Guidance: Ultrasound guidance is recommended to optimize delivery of the PRP to the exact location of the rotator cuff injury.

It is important to note that PRP protocols are not yet standardized, and the best approach may depend on the specific condition and the experience of the treating physician.

Quote from a Landmark Study

As noted by researchers Hamid and Sazlina in their 2021 landmark systematic review and meta-analysis, "PRP injection is a safe and effective intervention for long-term pain control and shoulder function in patients with rotator cuff disorders."

This statement highlights the promise of PRP as a regenerative treatment that may offer more than just symptom relief—it may support the actual healing of damaged shoulder tissues.

PRP for Shoulder Osteoarthritis: Evidence & Outcomes

Clinical evidence supports the use of platelet-rich plasma (PRP) injections as a non-operative treatment for glenohumeral joint (GHJ) osteoarthritis (OA), offering meaningful improvements in both pain and function. A large retrospective analysis involving patients with chondral damage in a major joint (including the shoulder) found sustained improvement in pain and functional scores up to 12 months after treatment. These benefits were seen across OA severities, although patients with lower-grade OA had better absolute outcomes. Multiple injections spaced 3–4 weeks apart were associated with superior results, especially in more active individuals.

PRP may not halt disease progression definitively, but studies suggest potential chondroprotective effects, largely due to its ability to inhibit matrix metalloproteinases, which are responsible for cartilage matrix degradation. By reducing catabolic activity and inflammation, PRP may help preserve existing cartilage and delay glenohumeral OA progression. Furthermore, some experimental data support a synergistic benefit when PRP is combined with hyaluronic acid (HA), with one study reporting significantly greater pain and function improvements at 1 year compared to HA alone.

A clinical series evaluating 45 shoulders with radiographic glenohumeral OA found that patients with less joint space loss had superior global improvement and joint preservation compared to those with near-complete joint space loss. Furthermore, those with less joint space loss were more likely to avoid joint replacement at 2 years. SANE and DASH scores improved at 6 months and were sustained for years, with some patients maintaining functional benefits up to 8 years.

Multiple randomized controlled trials (RCTs) and clinical studies have compared the efficacy of platelet-rich plasma (PRP) with hyaluronic acid (HA) and corticosteroid (CS) injections in the management of glenohumeral joint osteoarthritis (GHJ OA). A 2022 double-blind RCT involving 70 patients with GHJ OA found no significant difference in pain or function between ultrasound-guided injections of leukocyte-poor PRP and HA at any point over 12 months. However, both groups experienced statistically significant improvements in SPADI, ASES, and NRS scores starting at 1–2 months, regardless of OA severity.

Other studies have evaluated PRP versus steroid injection. A randomized controlled trial compared a single intra-articular injection of PRP versus triamcinolone acetate in 50 patients with mild to moderate GHJ OA, and found that both groups improved, but PRP demonstrated greater and more sustained functional and pain reduction at 3 months. This study concluded that while steroids may offer earlier relief, PRP's regenerative effects support its superiority for moderate OA.

A systematic review also supports this view, rating the evidence as Level I for PRP over steroids and equal to hyaluronic acid for mid-stage OA.

Importantly, PRP injections are generally safe when prepared and administered appropriately. Across controlled trials, adverse effects were minimal—primarily mild and transient, such as local discomfort. Side effects occurred in about 3% of patients, and no serious adverse events were reported in regulated settings.

In summary, PRP offers safe, moderate-to-sustained improvements in pain and function for glenohumeral joint OA, particularly with multiple injections and in less advanced disease. While direct cartilage regeneration remains unproven, PRP may reduce catabolic signaling and delay structural decline. Further high-quality, long-term RCTs with imaging and biomarker analysis are needed to define PRP's role as a disease-modifying agent in shoulder OA. PRP is at least as effective as HA and may offer longer-lasting benefits than steroids, particularly in moderate glenohumeral joint OA, likely due to its regenerative rather than anti-inflammatory mechanism of action.

Acromioclavicular (AC) joint pathologies are a common cause of shoulder pain, with AC joint osteoarthritis being the most frequently encountered condition.

In a pilot study examining PRP for patients with acromioclavicular joint (ACJ) arthritis unresponsive to exercise and NSAIDs for at least 2 months, 1 mL of PRP was injected directly into the AC joint. Thirteen patients were followed for an average of 8 months, with outcomes assessed using the Constant Score at 1, 3, and 6 months.

- The mean pre-injection Constant Score was 45. At 1 month, the mean score improved to a statistically significant value of 69. At 3 months, the score increased further to a statistically significant value of 81. By 6 months, the score reached 89, showing continued improvement, although this final change was not statistically significant.

While limited by a small sample size and lack of a control group, the study supports clinically meaningful functional improvement after PRP injection in AC joint arthritis. The authors conclude that PRP is a promising treatment for primary AC joint arthritis, although larger randomized controlled trials are recommended to further evaluate its efficacy.

PRP for Bursitis, Labral Tears, and Frozen Shoulder

PRP for Subacromial Bursitis

Subacromial bursitis is a condition involving fluid distension of the bursa in the shoulder from inflammation and irritation, often due to an underlying rotator cuff disorder. Early studies suggest that PRP injections may help reduce subacromial inflammation and irritation and improve symptoms:

- A study with 100 patients compared PRP to corticosteroid injections and found that the PRP group had greater long-term pain relief, measured by VAS (Visual Analog Scale).
- Another small trial with 67 patients showed that those receiving leukocyte-rich PRP experienced significantly better pain relief and shoulder movement than those who received physical therapy alone.
- While another study with 60 patients showed that corticosteroids worked faster in the first week, PRP provided more sustained relief over time.

These findings suggest PRP might be a helpful injection option for those with subacromial bursitis.

PRP for Labral Tears

The labrum is a ring of cartilage that helps to stabilize the shoulder. Labral tears are common in athletes and people who perform overhead activities. PRP use in labral tears is quite limited:

- A small case series followed two patients with glenoid labral tears who were treated with PRP injections. Both patients reported lower pain and some return of shoulder function, though the sample size is too small to draw strong conclusions.

- A review conducted by WorkSafeBC reported that PRP might reduce pain when injected near labral injuries, but current evidence is limited, and more studies are needed.

In summary, PRP for labral tears is promising but not yet well established. Further research is needed to determine the efficacy and optimal PRP protocol for shoulder labral tears.

PRP for Frozen Shoulder

Frozen shoulder, or adhesive capsulitis, involves shoulder pain and stiffness from shoulder capsule fibrosis that gradually develops, often for unknown reasons. Morbidity and dysfunction from this condition can sometimes last over a year. PRP has emerged as a potential treatment that can quicken the recovery from frozen shoulder:

- A meta-analysis of 1024 patients found that PRP was significantly more effective than other treatments (including steroids and physical therapy) in reducing pain and improving range of motion.
- Multiple studies (with sample sizes ranging from 60 to over 1,100 patients) showed that people receiving PRP had:

    Greater gains in shoulder movement (especially in abduction and flexion),

    Significant reductions in VAS pain scores,

    Improved functional scores on the SPADI (Shoulder Pain and Disability Index).

- One study of 66 patients showed that PRP worked just as well as steroid injections up to 6 months, but long-term (> 6 months), PRP was significantly better in all parameters.

Altogether, the evidence suggests that PRP may help reduce pain and support a faster recovery in frozen shoulder.

Key Takeaway Callout Box

What the Research Shows About PRP in the Shoulder:

- **Bursitis**: PRP offers longer-lasting pain relief than steroids in some studies.
- **Labral Tears**: Limited data—small studies show potential, but more research is needed.
- **Frozen Shoulder**: Evidence supports PRP for faster recovery, less pain, and better shoulder motion.

Study Results Summary

Strong: Meta-analyses, large RCTs (≥100 patients)

Moderate: Smaller controlled studies (30–99 patients)

Limited: Pilot, case series, or <30 patients

Table 5.1 Summary of Clinical Evidence for PRP in Common Shoulder Conditions

Condition	Study Name / Year	Number of Patients	PRP Type Used	Outcome Metrics	Evidence
Rotator Cuff Injury	Large Prospective Study	132	Not specified	Improved ASES, VAS, function, satisfaction	[illegible]
Rotator Cuff Injury	Meta-analysis (multiple studies)	>550	LR-PRP & LP-PRP	↓ Pain, ↑ shoulder function vs dry needling/physio	[illegible]
Tendinopathy	Ultrasound-guided PRP Study	30	Not specified	Short-term improvements in pain and function	[illegible]
Partial RCT	Systematic Review (Dakkak et al., 2021)	518	Not specified	46% improvement in pain and function vs conservative treatment	[illegible]
Full/Partial Tears	Large Study on Non-operative Treatment	641	Not specified	Significantly better shoulder function with PRP	[illegible]
Shoulder Arthritis (GHJ OA)	Retrospective Analysis	Large	Not specified	VAS ↓ from 5.4 to 3; SANE ↑ from 58.7 to ~78	[illegible]
Shoulder Arthritis	2022 Double-blind RCT (JBJS Journal)	70	LP-PRP	PRP + HA: significant ASES, SPADI, NRS gains	[illegible]
Shoulder Arthritis	Egyptian RCT (Menoufia University)	50	Not specified	PRP > steroid at 3 months (WOOS, VAS)	[illegible]
Shoulder Arthritis	Radiographic Cohort Study	45	Not specified	Joint preservation: 93.3%; sustained SANE/DASH gains	[illegible]
AC Joint Arthritis	Pilot Study (Double-spin method)	33 pts / 39 shoulders	Not specified	Constant Score ↑ from 45 → 89 over 6 months	[illegible]
Bursitis	RCT vs corticosteroids	100	Not specified	Longer-lasting VAS relief vs steroids	[illegible]
Bursitis	Small Trial	67	LR-PRP	Better pain and movement vs physical therapy	[illegible]
Labral Tears	Case Series + WorkSafeBC Review	2	Not specified	↓ Pain, some function gain; limited evidence	[illegible]
Frozen Shoulder	Meta-analysis	1024	Not specified	PRP > steroids/PT in pain relief and ROM	[illegible]
Frozen Shoulder	Multiple studies	60–1,100	Not specified	↑ ROM, ↓ VAS, improved SPADI	[illegible]

Future Research & What's on the Horizon

PRP has shown encouraging results for shoulder conditions, but researchers are still working to better understand the optimal PRP protocol, which may vary for each condition.

Ongoing and Upcoming Studies

Several clinical trials are underway to compare PRP to other treatments like steroid injections or surgery, and to explore whether PRP improves healing when used in addition to surgeries like a rotator cuff repair. Researchers are also studying whether different types of PRP—such as leukocyte-rich or leukocyte-poor—lead to better outcomes depending on the injury.

What We Still Don't Know

There are important questions that future research aims to answer:

- What is the ideal platelet dosage of PRP for shoulder conditions?
- Which shoulder conditions are better to use leukocyte-rich or leukocyte-poor PRP?
- Does platelet-poor plasma have a role in any shoulder conditions?

Answering these questions will help make PRP even more effective and personalized.

The Bigger Picture: Orthobiologics

PRP is part of a growing field called **orthobiologics**—treatments made from the body's natural materials to help treat and heal injuries. As this field expands, patients may have access to more advanced, targeted biologic options such as peptides, proteins, and stem cell treatments in the near future.

Key Takeaways

Summary Points

- PRP has shown promising results across a variety of shoulder conditions, including rotator cuff disorders, glenohumeral joint osteoarthritis, subacromial bursitis, AC joint arthritis, labral tears, and frozen shoulder.
- For rotator cuff disorders, both tendinopathies and partial tears respond well to PRP, with studies showing significant improvements in pain, shoulder function, and patient satisfaction.
- In glenohumeral osteoarthritis, PRP offers moderate to sustained relief of pain and functional impairment. It may also help delay joint replacement in early-stage disease.
- Subacromial bursitis responds favorably to PRP, with longer-lasting pain relief than corticosteroids in some trials.
- While shoulder labral tear data remains limited, early reports suggest PRP may reduce pain and support healing.
- Frozen shoulder has strong supporting evidence for PRP, with improvements in range of motion, pain reduction, and functional scores comparable to steroids but with fewer side effects.

Clinical Reassurance

- PRP is supported by a growing body of high-level evidence, including meta-analyses and randomized controlled trials, especially for conditions like rotator cuff tendinopathy, moderate glenohumeral osteoarthritis, and frozen shoulder.

- When properly prepared and administered, PRP has a strong safety profile, with minimal adverse events reported in controlled settings.
- Although protocols vary across studies, the consistent trend toward pain relief, functional gains, and improved quality of life underscores PRP's value in musculoskeletal care.

Looking Ahead

In the next chapter, we'll walk you through what to expect when preparing for your own PRP treatment—including how to plan your schedule, set realistic expectations, and optimize your outcomes with post-injection care strategies.

Bibliography

Blanchard, E., Harvi, J., Vasudevan, J., & Swanson, R. L., 2nd. (2023). Platelet-rich plasma for adhesive capsulitis: A systematic review. *Cureus, 15*(10), Article e46580. https://doi.org/10.7759/cureus.46580

Casa, D. J., Clarkson, P. M., & Roberts, W. O. (2005). American College of Sports Medicine roundtable on hydration and physical activity. *Current Sports Medicine Reports, 4*(4), 115–127. https://doi.org/10.1097/01.csmr.0000306194.67241.76

Dadgostar, H., Fahimipour, F., Pahlevan Sabagh, A., Araghi, A., Arasteh, P., & Maftoon, M. (2021). Corticosteroids or platelet-rich plasma injections for rotator cuff tendinopathy: A randomized clinical trial study. *Journal of Orthopaedic Surgery and Research, 16*, Article 333. https://doi.org/10.1186/s13018-021-02470-x

Dakkak, M., Saleem, A., Patel, D., Yeager, M., Oliveira, L., Gilot, G., & Spindler, K. P. (2024). A systematic review of randomized control trials looking at functional improvement of rotator cuff partial thickness tears following platelet-rich-plasma injection: A comparison of glenohumeral joint vs. subacromial bursa vs. intratendinous injection locations. *JSES International, 8*(3), 464–471. https://doi.org/10.1016/j.jseint.2024.01.003

Gupta, G. K., Shekhar, S., Haque, Z. U., Halder, S., Manjhi, A. K., & Rai, A. (2022). Comparison of the efficacy of platelet-rich plasma (PRP) and local corticosteroid injection in periarthritis shoulder: A Prospective, Randomized, Open, Blinded End-Point (PROBE) study. *Cureus*, *14*(9), Article e29253. https://doi.org/10.7759/cureus.29253

Hamid, M. S. A., & Sazlina, S. G. (2021). Platelet-rich plasma for rotator cuff tendinopathy: A systematic review and meta-analysis. *PLoS ONE*, *16*(5), Article e0251111. https://doi.org/10.1371/journal.pone.0251111

Haider, S. I., Awais, M. Z., & Iqbal, M. T. (2022). Role of platelet-rich plasma in the treatment of adhesive capsulitis: A prospective cohort study. *Cureus*, *14*(10), Article e30542. https://doi.org/10.7759/cureus.30542

Harna, B., Gupta, V., Arya, S., Jeyaraman, N., Rajendran, L. R., Jeyaraman, M., Gangadaran, P., Khanna, M., Hong, C. M., & Ahn, B. C. (2022). Current role of intra-articular injections of platelet-rich plasma in adhesive capsulitis of shoulder: A systematic review. *Bioengineering*, *10*(1), Article 21. https://doi.org/10.3390/bioengineering10010021

Hewavithana, P. B., Wettasinghe, M. C., Hettiarachchi, G., Ratnayaka, M., Suraweera, H., Wickramasinghe, N. D., & Kumarasiri, P. V. R. (2024). Effectiveness of single intra-bursal injection of platelet-rich plasma against corticosteroid under ultrasonography guidance for shoulder impingement syndrome: A randomized clinical trial. *Skeletal Radiology*, *53*(1), 51–58. https://doi.org/10.1007/s00256-023-04373-w

Ibrahim, D. H., El-Gazzar, N. M., El-Saadany, H. M., & El-Khouly, R. M. (2019). Ultrasound-guided injection of platelet rich plasma versus corticosteroid for treatment of rotator cuff tendinopathy: Effect on shoulder pain, disability, range of motion and ultrasonographic findings. *The Egyptian Rheumatologist*, *41*(2), 157–161. https://doi.org/10.1016/j.ejr.2018.06.004

Kirschner, J. S., Cheng, J., Creighton, A., Santiago, K., Hurwitz, N., Dundas, Mark., Beatty, N., Kingsbury, D., Konin, G., Abutalib, Z., & Chang, R. (2022). Efficacy of ultrasound-guided glenohumeral joint injections of leukocyte-poor platelet-rich plasma versus hyaluronic acid in the treatment of glenohumeral osteoarthritis: A randomized, double-blind controlled trial. *Clinical Journal of Sport Medicine*, *32*(6), 558–566. https://doi.org/10.1097/JSM.0000000000001029

Lin, H. W., Tam, K. W., Liou, T. H., Rau, C. L., Huang, S. W., & Hsu, T. H. (2023). Efficacy of platelet-rich plasma injection on range of motion, pain, and disability in patients with adhesive capsulitis: A systematic review and meta-analysis. *Archives of Physical Medicine and Rehabilitation*, *104*(12), 2109–2122. https://doi.org/10.1016/j.apmr.2023.03.032

Lum, Z. C., Guntupalli, L., & Huish, E. G. (2023). Outcomes of platelet rich plasma injections in the adhesive capsulitis of the shoulder. *Journal of Orthopaedics, 48*, 42–46. https://doi.org/10.1016/j.jor.2023.11.031

Maughan, R. J., & Griffin, J. (2003). Caffeine ingestion and fluid balance: A review. *Journal of Human Nutrition and Dietetics, 16*(6), 411–420. https://doi.org/10.1046/j.1365-277X.2003.00477.x

McEwen, B. J. (2010). The influence of diet and nutrients on platelet function. *Seminars in Thrombosis and Hemostasis, 36*(2), 126–136. https://doi.org/10.1055/s-0030-1251496

Montagnino, J., Kaufman, M. W., Shetty, M., Centeno, C., & Fredericson, M. (2025). Optimizing orthobiologic therapies with exercise, diet, and supplements. *PM&R*. Advance online publication. https://doi.org/10.1002/pmrj.13320

Pretorius, J., Habash, M., Ghobrial, B., Alnajjar, R., & Ellanti, P. (2023). Current status and advancements in platelet-rich plasma therapy. *Cureus, 15*(10), Article e30099.

Prodromos, C. C. (n.d.). *PRP injection of the arthritic glenohumeral joint is safe, effective, and avoids joint replacement in many patients at 2–8 year follow-up*. The Prodromos Stem Cell Institute. Retrieved June 20, 2025, from https://www.thepsci.com/prp-injection-of-the-arthritic-glenohumeral-joint.html

Prodromos, C. C., Finkle, S., Prodromos, A., Chen, J. L., Schwartz, A., & Wathen, L. (2021). Treatment of rotator cuff tears with platelet rich plasma: A prospective study with 2 year follow-up. *BMC Musculoskeletal Disorders, 22*(1), Article 499. https://doi.org/10.1186/s12891-021-04288-4

Raja, C., Sudhakar, T., Jambukeswaran, P. S. T., Ugeneshwaran, M., & Manivannan, A. G. (2020). PRP in acromio-clavicular joint arthritis – A prospective analysis. *IP International Journal of Orthopaedic Rheumatology, 6*(2), 80–83.

Rossi, L. A., Brandariz, R., Gorodischer, T., Camino, P., Piuzzi, N., Tanoira, I., & Ranalletta, M. (2024). Subacromial injection of platelet-rich plasma provides greater improvement in pain and functional outcomes compared to corticosteroids at 1-year follow-up: A double-blinded randomized controlled trial. *Journal of Shoulder and Elbow Surgery, 33*(12), 2563–2571. https://doi.org/10.1016/j.jse.2024.06.012

Rossi, L. A., Piuzzi, N. S., & Shapiro, S. A. (2020). Glenohumeral osteoarthritis: The role for orthobiologic therapies: Platelet-rich plasma and cell therapies. *JBJS Reviews, 8*(2), Article e0075. https://doi.org/10.2106/JBJS.RVW.19.00075

Rossi, L. A., Piuzzi, N. S., Tanoira, I., Brandariz, R., Huespe, I., & Ranalletta, M. (2023). Subacromial platelet-rich plasma injections produce significantly worse improvement in functional outcomes in patients with partial supraspinatus tears than in patients with isolated tendinopathy. *Arthroscopy: The Journal of Arthroscopic & Related Surgery, 39*(9), 2000–2008. https://doi.org/10.1016/j.arthro.2023.03.019

Saif, D. S., Serag, D. M., & El Tabl, M. A. (2019). Comparative study between platelet-rich plasma injection and steroid injection in mild–moderate shoulder osteoarthritis and their relation to quality of life. *Egyptian Rheumatology and Rehabilitation, 46*(1), 55–61.

Schwitzguébel, A., Corzo, A. H., Theodoridou, E., & Lädermann, A. (2025). Platelet-rich plasma treatment for large joint osteoarthritis: Retrospective study highlighting a possible treatment protocol with long-lasting stimulation of the joint with an adequate dose of platelets. *BMC Musculoskeletal Disorders, 26*(1), Article 412. https://doi.org/10.1186/s12891-025-08663-3

Singh, S., Agarwal, P., & Sharma, A. (2025). One year results of intraarticular platelet rich plasma in adhesive capsulitis of shoulder. Journal of Orthopaedic Reports, 4(1), 100532. https://doi.org/10.1016/j.jorep.2024.100532

Useros, N. R., Nova, E., Zapatera, B., Gheorghe, A., Olivares, M., & Marcos, A. (2015). Influence of alcohol consumption on hydration status in healthy adults. *Nutrición Hospitalaria.*

Vander Kraats, R., & Doss, A. (2012). Glenoid labral tear: Follow up case series on ultrasound guided autologous platelet rich plasma in conjunction with a progressive rehabilitation program. *F1000Research*, *1*, Article 68. https://doi.org/10.12688/f1000research.1-68.v1

Violi, F., Pignatelli, P., & Basili, S. (2010). Nutrition, supplements, and vitamins in platelet function and bleeding. *Circulation*, *121*(8), 1033–1042.

WorkSafeBC Evidence-Based Practice Group, & Martin, C. W. (2024). *Effectiveness of platelet-rich plasma therapy (PRP) in treating shoulder labral tears.* WorkSafeBC Evidence-Based Practice Group.

Xu, W., & Xue, Q. (2021). Application of platelet-rich plasma in arthroscopic rotator cuff repair: A systematic review and meta-analysis. *Orthopaedic Journal of Sports Medicine*, *9*(7), Article 23259671211016847. https://doi.org/10.1177/23259671211016847

Yu, S., Hu, R., Feng, H., & Huang, D. (2023). Efficacy of platelet-rich plasma injection in the treatment of frozen shoulder: A systematic review and meta-analysis. *Journal of Back and Musculoskeletal Rehabilitation*, *36*(3), 551–564. https://doi.org/10.3233/BMR-220034

Zhang, W. B., Ma, Y. L., Lu, F. L., Guo, HR., Song, H., & Hu, Y. M. (2024). The clinical efficacy and safety of platelet-rich plasma on frozen shoulder: A systematic review and meta-analysis of randomized controlled trials. *BMC Musculoskeletal Disorders*, *25*(1), Article 718. https://doi.org/10.1186/s12891-024-07629-1

Zhu, P., Wang, Z., Li, H., & Cai, Y. (2022). Platelet-rich plasma injection in non-operative treatment of partial-thickness rotator cuff tears: A systematic review and meta-analysis. *Journal of Rehabilitation Medicine*, *54*, Article jrm00312. https://doi.org/10.2340/jrm.v54.1434

Ziroglu, N., & Şahbaz, Y. (2024). Clinical effects of additional platelet-rich plasma application to exercise therapy in patients with subacromial impingement syndrome: A double-blind randomized controlled trial. *Orthopaedic Journal of Sports Medicine*, *12*(10), Article 23259671241276368. https://doi.org/10.1177/23259671241276368

CHAPTER 6

Who is a Candidate for PRP?

Author: Gayan Poovendran

Platelet-Rich Plasma (PRP) therapy harnesses the healing potential of your own blood to treat orthopedic conditions. It is most effective when used in the right clinical context. The ideal candidate profile depends on both the nature of the shoulder pathology and the overall health status of the patient.

Ideal Candidates

Mild to Moderate Shoulder Pathology

PRP has shown promise in treating conditions such as partial-thickness rotator cuff tears, chronic tendinosis, early adhesive capsulitis (frozen shoulder), subacromial bursitis, and early-stage glenohumeral osteoarthritis (Kellgren-Lawrence grade I–II). In these cases, tissue integrity is preserved enough for biological signaling to influence healing. Numerous studies have demonstrated improved pain and functional scores in these populations, particularly when PRP is administered under image guidance.

Case Example: A 58-year-old recreational swimmer presented with chronic supraspinatus tendinosis and subacromial pain despite 3 months of physical therapy. Ultrasound-guided PRP was injected into the affected tendon, followed by a structured rehab protocol. Within 6 weeks, the patient reported reduced night pain and was able to resume swimming without discomfort.

Athletes Seeking Non-Surgical Recovery

Athletes, especially those in overhead or contact sports, often seek alternatives to surgery. PRP can accelerate healing and reduce downtime without violating anti-doping regulations. When paired with rest and structured rehabilitation, athletes may resume activity sooner than with conventional care alone.

Case Example: A 25-year-old National Football League athlete with a partial rotator cuff tear declined surgical intervention. After PRP treatment and a modified training schedule with tailored physical therapy, the patient returned to pre-injury activity within 10 weeks with full function restored.

Patients with Incomplete Response to Conservative Care

If standard non-surgical therapies (physical therapy, activity modification, oral medications) have failed to produce meaningful improvement after 6–12 weeks, PRP can offer a minimally invasive next step. It is often used as a biological adjunct to bridge the gap before considering surgical options.

Who May Not Be a Candidate

Advanced Degeneration or Structural Irreparability

Patients with full-thickness rotator cuff tears, retracted tendons, advanced osteoarthritis (KL grade III–IV), or structural defects requiring surgical repair are unlikely to benefit significantly from PRP alone. In these scenarios, the mechanical architecture of the joint is too compromised for PRP biological treatments to provide adequate relief.

Case Example: A 70-year-old patient with severe shoulder arthritis and limited range of motion underwent PRP injection with minimal improvement. The patient ultimately required shoulder replacement for meaningful functional recovery.

Contraindicated Medical Conditions

Patients with active systemic infections, platelet or bleeding disorders, poorly controlled diabetes (HbA1c > 8.0%), or current cancer/chemotherapy may not be suitable candidates. These conditions impair healing or pose increased risks from the injection process.

Evidence Highlights:

- A 2021 RCT in *The American Journal of Sports Medicine* involving 90 patients with partial rotator cuff tears showed significantly greater improvements in ASES and Constant scores at 6 months post-PRP compared to saline.
- A 2022 meta-analysis in *Arthroscopy* covering 13 studies found PRP significantly reduced pain and improved function in adhesive capsulitis compared to placebo or corticosteroid injections.
- A 2023 review in the *Journal of Shoulder Elbow Surgery* concluded that PRP may delay progression in early-stage glenohumeral arthritis when used with physical therapy and anti-inflammatory measures.

Medications & Supplements to Avoid

Because PRP therapy relies on the activation and function of your body's own platelets, certain medications and supplements can significantly interfere with its effectiveness.

This section explains which agents should be paused before your procedure, why they matter, and how to safely prepare with your healthcare team.

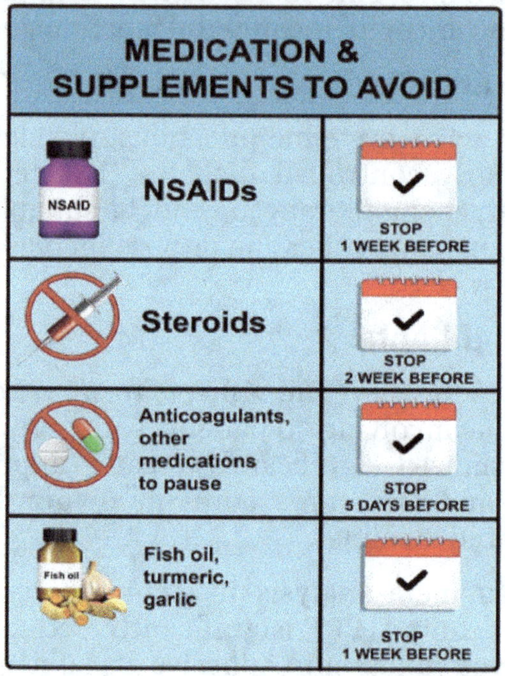

Figure 6.1 Common Medications and Supplements to Avoid Before PRP Treatment

This infographic highlights medications and supplements that may be temporarily discontinued before PRP therapy, including nonsteroidal anti-inflammatory drugs (NSAIDs), corticosteroids, certain anticoagulants, and selected dietary supplements. Because these agents may influence platelet function, inflammation, or bleeding risk, patients should always follow the specific instructions provided by their treating physician regarding medication management before a PRP procedure.

Why This Matters

Platelets are more than just clotting cells—they contain powerful growth factors and signaling proteins that initiate the healing cascade. For PRP to work, these platelets must be collected in their functional form and allowed to activate properly once injected into the injured area.

Medications or supplements that impair platelet aggregation, reduce inflammation artificially, or thin the blood can:

- Reduce the concentration of growth factors released at the target site
- Prolong bleeding at the injection site
- Delay or blunt the healing response
- Lead to complications such as bruising or post-injection inflammation

Therefore, understanding what to stop—and when—is a key part of successful PRP treatment.

NSAIDs (Non-Steroidal Anti-Inflammatory Drugs)

Examples: Ibuprofen (Advil, Motrin), Naproxen (Aleve), Diclofenac (Voltaren), Celecoxib (Celebrex)

NSAIDs are among the most common over-the-counter medications used for pain and inflammation. However, they inhibit COX enzymes (cyclooxygenase-1 and -2), which are critical for platelet activation and the early stages of tissue repair. When taken around the time of a PRP injection,

NSAIDs can significantly reduce the efficacy of the treatment.

Clinical Insight:

A 2020 *in vitro* study published in *The Journal of Translational Medicine* showed that platelet-derived growth factor (PDGF) and transforming growth factor-beta (TGF-β) release was significantly reduced in patients who had taken NSAIDs in the 5 days prior to PRP draw.

Recommendations:

- Discontinue NSAIDs **at least 5–7 days before** your PRP appointment.
- Avoid restarting NSAIDs for **4–6 weeks after** the injection unless instructed by your physician.
- Consider using acetaminophen (Tylenol) for pain relief if needed, as it does not interfere with platelet function.

Patient Tip: Many combination cold or allergy medications contain NSAIDs—always check labels.

Corticosteroids

Examples: Oral prednisone, methylprednisolone; injected corticosteroids (e.g., Kenalog, cortisone)

Corticosteroids are potent anti-inflammatory medications that can reduce pain, but they also suppress immune cell signaling and collagen synthesis. If taken shortly before a PRP injection, steroids may inhibit the controlled inflammation PRP is meant to create, undermining the therapeutic intent.

Timing Matters:

- If you've had a **steroid injection in your shoulder** recently, your physician will likely delay PRP until **6–8 weeks have passed**.

- Oral steroids should ideally be avoided for **at least 2–4 weeks** prior to PRP unless medically necessary.

Why This Is Important:

PRP works by triggering a localized healing response. Steroids do the opposite—they suppress that response. Administering PRP too soon after a steroid shot may negate the regenerative effects.

Patient Scenario: A 65-year-old patient received a cortisone injection for rotator cuff pain but continued to struggle with limited motion and opted for PRP. Because the steroid was injected just 2 weeks prior, the PRP procedure was scheduled for 6 weeks out to avoid a suppressed healing response.

Anticoagulants and Antiplatelet Medications

Examples:

- Anticoagulants: Warfarin (Coumadin), Apixaban (Eliquis), Rivaroxaban (Xarelto), Dabigatran (Pradaxa)
- Antiplatelets: Clopidogrel (Plavix), high-dose aspirin (>81 mg/day)

These medications are prescribed to reduce the risk of clotting in patients with heart disease, atrial fibrillation, deep vein thrombosis, or a history of stroke. However, they also increase the risk of bleeding or bruising from any injection procedure and may affect clot formation around the PRP site.

What to Do:

- Never stop a prescribed blood thinner without first consulting the physician who manages your cardiac or vascular care.
- Your PRP provider **may** coordinate with your

cardiologist to pause these medications **3–5 days before** treatment if it is deemed safe.

Aspirin:

- Low-dose (81 mg) aspirin is sometimes allowed to continue, depending on your medical history.
- High-dose aspirin (>325 mg/day) should be stopped **5–7 days prior** to your procedure. However, discussion with your provider prior to stopping any medication is important.

Supplements with Blood-Thinning Effects

Many common over-the-counter supplements and natural remedies have mild anticoagulant effects that can increase bleeding or interfere with platelet aggregation.

Supplements to Pause:

- **Fish Oil/Omega-3s**: Often used for cardiovascular health but known to reduce platelet stickiness.
- **Turmeric/Curcumin**: Anti-inflammatory, but can inhibit platelet aggregation.
- **Ginkgo Biloba**: Popular for memory support, but has anticoagulant properties.
- **Vitamin E**: In high doses, it can thin the blood and impair clotting.
- **Garlic (especially in concentrated pill form)**

Note: While dietary sources of omega-3s (like salmon and walnuts) are encouraged for their anti-inflammatory benefits, concentrated omega-3 supplements (like fish oil pills) should be paused due to their blood-thinning effect.

Recommendations:

- Stop these supplements **7–10 days prior** to your injection.
- Inform your provider about any herbal blends, teas, or powders you are taking regularly.
- If you are using multiple supplements, bring a full list to your pre-procedure consultation.

Patient Note: Even "natural" products can have powerful effects on your body. The fact that a supplement is sold without a prescription does not mean it is benign in the context of a precision procedure like PRP.

Final Thoughts

The medications and supplements you take every day may seem unrelated to your joint health, but they can dramatically impact your body's response to PRP therapy. A short pause—under medical supervision—can make a measurable difference in your results.

If you're unsure whether a particular medication or supplement is safe to continue, don't guess—ask your provider. Clear communication and proactive planning are essential for maximizing your outcome.

Optimizing Platelet Function and Healing Potential

Because PRP is derived from your own blood, the quality of the treatment depends directly on your personal health. In the days leading up to your procedure, simple adjustments in hydration, nutrition, rest, and stress management can meaningfully enhance the effectiveness of your PRP injection. Think of it as "prepping the soil" before planting the seed.

Hydration

Plasma—the fluid portion of your blood—is essential for PRP

separation. Being dehydrated can reduce plasma volume and limit the concentration of usable platelets.

- Aim to **keep well hydrated**. Aim for **2 liters (8 cups) or 64 ounces** of water daily, starting at least **3 days** before your procedure; however, discussion with your provider is warranted.
- Avoid alcohol and excess caffeine, both of which dehydrate the body.
- A good hydration goal: pale yellow urine.

Tip: Start hydrating early in the day; front-loading fluids avoids late-night disruptions to sleep.

Sleep and Stress Management

Sleep deprivation and stress elevate **cortisol**, a hormone that can reduce platelet performance and impair healing. Recovery is a full-body process—and sleep plays a central role.

- Aim for **7–9 hours** of uninterrupted sleep each night.
- Avoid screens for an hour before bed and maintain a consistent bedtime.
- Incorporate light daily movement, breathing exercises, or mindfulness to lower stress levels.

Note: Well-rested patients tend to tolerate the procedure better and report fewer post-injection symptoms.

Anti-Inflammatory Nutrition

What you eat influences your body's internal inflammation and repair signals. An anti-inflammatory diet can enhance PRP's regenerative effects by creating a healing-friendly environment.

Foods to Prioritize:

- Omega-3 fats: salmon, walnuts, flaxseed
- Colorful produce: berries, spinach, carrots
- Collagen-supportive nutrients: citrus fruits, leafy greens, bone broth

Foods to Limit:

- Refined sugars and processed snacks
- Deep-fried foods and trans fats
- Excess alcohol and soda

Timing: Adopt this diet **at least 5–7 days prior** to your injection and continue it post-procedure to support recovery.

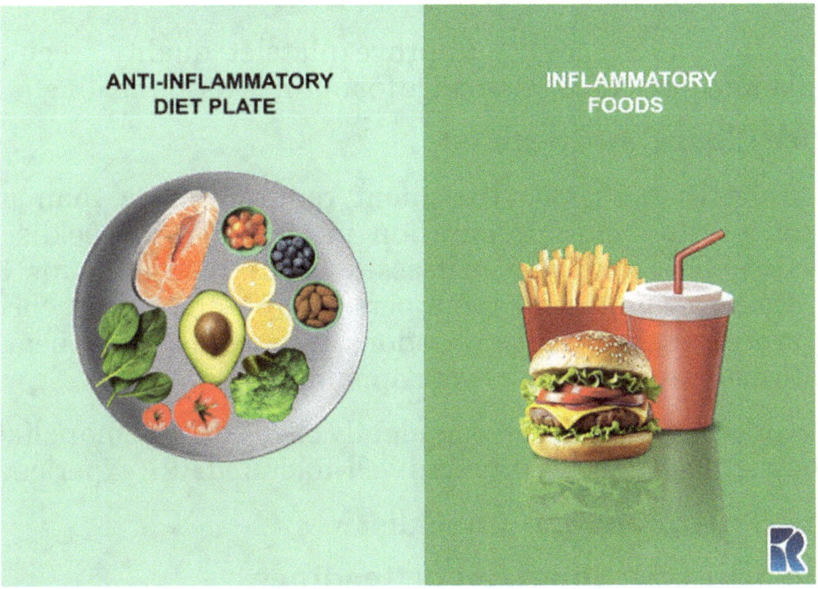

Figure 6.2 Dietary Choices That May Influence Inflammation and Tissue Recovery

This illustration contrasts foods commonly associated with an anti-inflammatory dietary pattern, including fruits, vegetables, fish, nuts, and healthy fats, with highly processed foods that may contribute to a pro-inflammatory state. Nutritional habits may influence overall health, recovery, and the body's response to injury and tissue repair processes.

Summary

Small, strategic changes can significantly influence how your body responds to PRP. Prioritize:

- Staying hydrated
- Sleeping well
- Managing stress
- Eating nutrient-dense, anti-inflammatory foods

Together, these habits improve platelet quality, regulate inflammation, and set the stage for optimal tissue healing.

PRP Eligibility Checklist

Platelet-Rich Plasma treatment requires more than just showing up—your preparation matters. This checklist is designed to help you self-assess your readiness for the procedure. Think of it as your personal pre-flight safety check: if any of these items raise questions or concerns, bring them up with your provider before your appointment.

The more items you can confidently check off, the more likely you are to have an effective and well-tolerated PRP experience.

Pre-Treatment Self-Checklist

Medication & Supplement Readiness

- I have not taken NSAIDs (e.g., ibuprofen, naproxen) in the last 7 days.

- I am not currently taking blood thinners OR have been cleared by my prescribing provider to pause them.
- I have not received a steroid injection in the treatment area within the past 6–8 weeks.

Health & Healing Capacity

- I have no active infections, fever, or illness.
- My blood sugar is well-controlled (if I have diabetes).
- I am well-hydrated and have increased my water intake in the past 3–5 days.
- I have been sleeping 7–9 hours per night and managing stress.
- I have been eating a nutrient-rich, anti-inflammatory diet for at least 5 days.

Mindset & Expectations

- I understand that PRP is **not** a quick fix and that promotion of healing is gradual.
- I am willing to follow my provider's post-procedure instructions (including physical therapy, rest, or temporary activity modification).
- I feel mentally prepared and optimistic about using my body's own healing potential.

What If I Can't Check Every Box?

Don't worry—**this checklist is a guide**, not a pass/fail exam. If you are unsure about a medication, have a health condition, or haven't quite nailed your sleep or diet yet, your provider can help you make a tailored plan. The goal is to give your body the best possible foundation for recovery.

Questions to Ask Your Physician

PRP therapy is a biologically driven treatment, but its success also depends on the skill, technique, and judgment of the provider. Choosing the right clinician and asking the right questions can make a significant difference in both your experience and your outcome.

Whether you're new to regenerative medicine or just doing your due diligence, this list will help you prepare for a productive consultation.

Questions to Ask During Your PRP Consultation

Experience & Technique

- How many PRP injections have you performed for shoulder conditions?
- Do you use **ultrasound and/or fluoroscopic guidance** to ensure precise placement of the injection?
- What is your training in regenerative or musculoskeletal medicine?

Treatment Details

- What PRP system do you use, and how does it compare to others?
- Do you customize the platelet concentration or volume based on my condition?
- Will you be drawing the blood and injecting it on the same day?

Integration with Rehab

- How do you coordinate PRP with physical therapy or post-treatment exercises?

- When should I resume regular activity or training after the injection?
- Do you recommend a specific physical therapist or rehab protocol?

Outcomes & Expectations

- What type of improvement can I reasonably expect, and over what time frame?
- What are your success rates with PRP in patients similar to me?
- What happens if PRP doesn't work—what are my next options?

What to Listen For

Your provider should be comfortable discussing the science behind PRP, the rationale for their technique, and their clinical results. Look for thoughtful answers, not vague promises. Beware of overly commercialized or one-size-fits-all approaches—true regenerative medicine is personalized.

Reminder: This is your body, your recovery, and your investment. You deserve clarity, transparency, and partnership.

Confidence & Mindset Before the Procedure

It's perfectly normal to feel a little anxious before trying something new—especially when it involves needles, your shoulder, and a treatment you may have only recently heard about. But PRP is not experimental anymore. It is evidence-based, widely practiced, and designed to work with your body—not against it.

This is not just another injection. It is a shift toward **biological healing**, using your own cells to repair and regenerate injured tissue. PRP does not mask pain like a steroid—it encourages real recovery over time.

That is why mindset matters.

Coming into your procedure with **realistic expectations** and a commitment to post-injection care (like physical therapy, hydration, and activity pacing) can make all the difference. Patients who trust the process, stay consistent, and stay engaged with their care team often see the strongest results.

Key Takeaways:

- PRP is not a quick fix—it's a gradual reboot for your body.
- Progress may come in phases: less pain, better motion, improved function.
- Your attitude, discipline, and optimism are powerful parts of the healing equation.

Bottom line: You're not just receiving a procedure. You're taking an active role in your recovery—and that is a bold, positive step forward.

Bibliography

Casa, D. J., Clarkson, P. M., & Roberts, W. O. (2005). American College of Sports Medicine roundtable on hydration and physical activity. *Current Sports Medicine Reports*, *4*(4), 115–127. https://doi.org/10.1097/01.csmr.0000306194.67241.76

Hamid, M. S. A., & Sazlina, S. G. (2021). Platelet-rich plasma for rotator cuff tendinopathy: A systematic review and meta-analysis. *PLoS ONE*, *16*(5), Article e0251111. https://doi.org/10.1371/journal.pone.0251111

Maughan, R. J., & Griffin, J. (2003). Caffeine ingestion and fluid balance: A review. *Journal of Human Nutrition and Dietetics*, *16*(6), 411–420. https://doi.org/10.1046/j.1365-277X.2003.00477.x

McEwen, B. J. (2010). The influence of diet and nutrients on platelet function. *Seminars in Thrombosis and Hemostasis*, *36*(2), 126–136. https://doi.org/10.1055/s-0030-1251496

Montagnino, J., Kaufman, M. W., Shetty, M., Centeno, C., & Fredericson, M. (2025). Optimizing orthobiologic therapies with exercise, diet, and supplements. *PM&R*. Advance online publication. https://doi.org/10.1002/pmrj.13320

Useros, N. R., Nova, E., Zapatera, B., Gheorghe, A., Olivares, M., & Marcos, A. (2015). Influence of alcohol consumption on hydration status in healthy adults. *Nutrición Hospitalaria*, *31*(6), 2686–2695.

https://doi.org/10.3305/nh.2015.31.6.8612

Violi, F., Pignatelli, P., & Basili, S. (2010). Nutrition, supplements, and vitamins in platelet function and bleeding. *Circulation*, *121*(8), 1033–1042.

CHAPTER 7

What to Expect After PRP Injections

Author: Prathap Jayaram

Due to the various uses of PRP for both tendon and joint pathology, patients' responses are highly variable following injection. Guidance following a procedure must be tailored to the condition and treatment. For example, patients' self-reported responses and rehabilitation may be different if PRP was used as an injectate for a knee joint injection versus an intra-tendinous injection for lateral epicondylitis. Despite the variability, the purpose of this chapter is to provide general guidance for providers and patients regarding what to expect following a PRP injection.

Immediate Aftercare: First 24 Hours

In the first 24 hours after the procedure, it is common to feel discomfort depending on the location of the injection. This is due to the acute inflammatory response to the tissue damage caused by the PRP injectate. However, the treated area is commonly numb in the first hour after the injection. This numbness can be due to the use of an anesthetic (i.e., lidocaine) at the site of the injection. After the numbing agent wears off, the patient may begin to feel a worsening of pain symptoms. The pain is due to inflammation in the area from the injection and the volume of the injection. The inflammation and volume can also lead to the body responding with soreness, swelling, warmth, redness, or stiffness. The reason for this inflammation is that the PRP acts on the body to stimulate healing. The symptoms may last for a day or two after the treatment.

Although there is no single standardized post-PRP protocols, there are several recommended modalities that are suggested to avoid so as not to have any interaction with the effects of the PRP. As the PRP is high in platelets, it is essential to avoid any medications that may diminish the impact of the injection. It is recommended to avoid NSAIDs, such as Aspirin (ASA), Aleve, Ibuprofen, and Diclofenac, for at least 24–48 hours after the injection. The reason for avoiding the use of NSAIDs is that they diminish the platelet function, which is key to the PRP's ability to treat patients. NSAIDs work to impair platelet function via the cyclooxygenase (COX)-1 and COX-2 inhibition. This anti-platelet effect has been demonstrated both *in vitro* and *in vivo*, thus leading to the conclusion that NSAIDs may negatively affect the proangiogenic and pro-inflammatory effects of PRP. Jayaram and colleagues in 2019 found that there were multiple diminished pro-inflammatory growth factors in arachidonic acid-activated PRP following 2 weeks of daily ASA use in men. Given these concerns, it is recommended to take Tylenol post-procedure instead of NSAIDs.

For patients experiencing post-procedural pain, there are numerous methods encouraged to reduce pain and improve overall comfort. Cryotherapy (Ice) may play a crucial role in pain management and analgesia following PRP injection. However, some argue that cryotherapy should not be used following PRP. The main theoretical risk of cryotherapy is the concern for reduced blood flow and inflammation at the site of intervention, which is essential for healing. There has been limited research supporting this concern. One study found that there is reduced blood flow within the first minute of cryotherapy to the Achilles tendon and then the return of normal circulation shortly after during recovery.

In addition to pain management, it is important that patients remain hydrated pre-procedurally as well as after the procedure. Pre-procedural hydration may allow for an easier blood draw. Additionally, after the blood draw, there may be feelings of light-headedness, which can be better managed with hydration. If desired, patients may engage in light activity. Normal, day-to-day activities are permitted as long as pain allows.

During the first 24 hours following the procedure, contact your provider if you have any questions.

Please contact your provider immediately if you find yourself with any concerning red flag symptoms. These include, but are not limited to, severe pain at the site of the injection, bleeding, signs of infection such as streaking, fever, chills, or excessive swelling. As the PRP is derived from your blood, there is no chance of an allergy or immune reaction. In the literature, reported complications are extremely rare. The main risks include local infection and pain at the injection site. While some redness and swelling are common after the procedure, if there is any progressive swelling, redness, or drainage, notify your provider immediately. If your symptoms are severe, you may be encouraged to go to the Emergency Room for an evaluation.

Recovery Timeline: When Will I Feel Better?

The central question for most patients is when they will begin to feel better, as well as feel the effects of the PRP post-injection. This process of recovering from the PRP injection can be broken up into 3 phases. These typical phases are the inflammatory flare phase, the proliferation phase, and the remodeling phase.

The first phase, the inflammatory phase, typically lasts the first 3 to 5 days following the injection. This phase is characterized by the body initiating the healing process by forming blood clots by aggregating platelets and thrombocytes in a fibrin network, thus "walling off" the injured site. This blood clot then acts as a barrier and helps to organize a temporary matrix needed for further cell migration events. During this time, the platelet plug then acts to secrete chemokines, or healing factors (e.g., platelet-derived growth factor [PDGF], fibrinogen, epidermal growth factor [EGF], and vascular endothelial growth factor [VEGF]), that lead to recruitment of macrophages, as well as fibroblasts, to the site of healing. This results in both debridement of the wound as well as formation of granulation tissue. Additionally, the secretion of chemokines increases the permeability of the blood vessels and allows more tissue nutrition while also providing the formation of granulation tissue necessary for the second stage. During this time, the patient may feel temporary inflammation and discomfort, as well as swelling, redness, and limited range of motion.

The second phase of healing, also referred to as the proliferation or granulation phase, typically lasts the first couple of weeks following injury. The phase is essential as the body begins forming the epithelial barrier, allowing the wound to begin to heal. This period of time is characterized by granulation tissue formation, collagen deposition, and angiogenesis around the surrounding bed of injury. Angiogenesis also provides a fresh supply of cells and nutrients to the injury site.

Initially, during this phase, fibroblasts will begin to synthesize collagen for the extracellular matrix. Earlier in the healing phase, collagen fibers tend to be randomly organized, and the matrix is composed of increasing amounts of type III collagen. As we move further from the procedure, newly deposited collagen fibers begin to be oriented along the direction of the force of the tendon.

During this time, there is found to be a gradual improvement. Patients may begin to feel pain relief and improvement in function. Acute post-procedure pain should begin to subside. Overall, patients may return to a similar level of pre-procedural symptoms.

The third and final phase, the remodeling phase, begins after the proliferation phase and typically lasts up to a year following PRP. The body works to remodel the new connective tissue that has grown. As the remodeling processes occur, mechanical stress can influence the process and promote increased tensile strength of the tissue. During this time, the preference shifts from deposition of type III collagen to an increased deposition of type 1 collagen. There are also a variety of cellular processes that occur with the emigration of cells and the apoptosis of fibroblasts. These inflammatory or endothelial cells lead to the formation of a scar. As a result, the inflammation continues to improve, leading to substantial pain relief, and the stronger treated area allows for greater stability and function. Patients can, however, continue to have intermittent symptoms during this period as the tissue continues to transition to scar formation.

Based on available data, there are general milestones that are expected to be reached in the post-procedural period. Given the number of varied pathologies PRP is used to treat, there is some variability in weekly goals. In general, the first week following PRP, the goal is relative rest. At this time, patients should avoid excess stress on the area of treatment. The patient's pain may typically peak in the first few days following the procedure and slowly begin to improve by the end of the first week. By the second week following the procedure, patients should generally start to have improved pain and may return to their baseline pre-procedural pain level. Patients should begin active range of motion and stretching programs. Patients should begin to slowly return to activities and begin a strengthening program by the second to third week following the procedure. As more time progresses, patients should continue to have greater improvement in both pain and function.

Post-Injection Care Recommendations

In most cases, following PRP, it is recommended to advise protected weight bearing for the first 48 hours following the injection. After the procedure, there is still a period where it is crucial not to put the body under unnecessary stress. Most randomized controlled trials have a period of, at a minimum, relative rest following injection. Levine and colleagues found that 35% of randomized-controlled trials examining intra-articular PRP for knee OA called for activity restriction. The timing of these restrictions varied from 1 day to 2 weeks. Early reduction in joint or tendon motion may additionally aid in reducing pain and swelling. Similarly, it is advised that patients avoid any activities or movements that provoke their pain. There is no set standard for immobilization following PRP. Recommendations in the literature range from immobilization and complete restriction of motion to only avoiding repetitive motion. If needed, crutches, a walking boot, or various bracing can be used to decrease stress on the joint or tendon. Regardless of the type of restrictions in the first couple of days following PRP, it is important to limit the duration of immobilization and initiate a general range of motion activities within a few days following injection.

Prolonged immobilization has been associated with both functional impairments and joint contractures.

Within 3–5 days following the procedure, it can be important for patients to incorporate and reintroduce gentle motion. There is no consensus regarding the optimal timing to initiate a gentle range of motion and stretching. As previously noted, there are a number of pathologies that PRP is used to treat. As such, intra-articular, intraosseous, and tendonous/ligamentous injections may require different periods of rest or activity modifications following PRP. Generally, it is advised that patients return to activity gradually and as tolerated. A recent review by Levine and colleagues in 2019 found that the majority of studies examining PRP for knee OA instructed patients to gradually return to stretching and activity as their pain allows. Overall, it is suggested that patients should limit any activity that causes their pain to increase to over a 3/10 pain level. Most protocols recommend that patients begin a form of physiotherapy and strengthening program around 1–2 weeks post-procedure. Although the timing of initiating strengthening may vary, patients undergoing intra-articular injection tend to initiate therapy and strengthening sooner than those undergoing intra-tendinous injections. During this time, rehabilitation should consist of a progressive strengthening program, focusing on isometric exercises in the beginning and eventually progressing to eccentric exercises.

Throughout the post-injection phases, it is essential to try to remain physically healthy as well as to avoid other triggers that can affect the PRP results. In order to optimize healing, it is best to avoid anything that may affect the healing and inflammatory cascade, including alcohol, smoking, or any inflammatory foods. These triggers can adversely affect the body's healing capabilities and limit recovery from the PRP inflammatory response. It may also decrease the full potential of the PRP in treating the target site. *In vitro*, it has been found that increased levels of alcohol consumption are linked to decreased platelet activation and aggregation, as well as reduced platelet response to thrombin and collagen. The same effect is found with smoking, as limiting smoking is seen to increase platelet aggregation. Due to this, a recent consensus statement recommends avoiding both alcohol and tobacco in the peri-procedural period. With a limit of these factors, it may allow the platelets to normalize their factor content and aggregation properties, which may be beneficial.

Checklist: Post-PRP Care Instructions

Following PRP injection, there are general guidelines that patients should follow in order to allow for optimization of the healing cascade and allow for the best pain and functional outcomes. Below is a checklist of recommended post-procedural care instructions. Both activity restriction and rehabilitation guidelines may vary depending on the type of tissue treated.

- Drink at least 64 ounces of water daily to maintain hydration
- Avoid anti-inflammatory medications such as Advil, Motrin, Ibuprofen, Aleve, Naproxen, and Meloxicam for at least 2 weeks after your procedure.
- Do not take hot baths or go to saunas during the first few days following your procedure.
- Do not consume alcoholic beverages for the first 7 days following your procedure.
- Avoid smoking.
- After 2–4 days, begin to incorporate increasing exercise and daily activities into your routine.

- After 2–4 weeks, it may be time to incorporate organized physical therapy into the program.
- Schedule follow-up appointments for approximately 6 weeks to see how you are doing and to ensure you are tracking well. This is also the time to ensure there are no adverse side effects from the PRP injection.

Common Patient Questions Post-PRP

As the field of orthobiologics continues to grow, patients seeking PRP may have questions regarding PRP and what the recovery following an injection may look like. Below are a few common questions that patients may ask their provider.

How long until I see improvement?

It is important to educate patients that the results of the PRP are gradual, especially compared to those of corticosteroid injections that provide immediate relief. It may take several months before improvement is seen. Overall, PRP, if effective, provides longer symptomatic relief than a corticosteroid injection, which typically loses efficacy by three months.

When can I return to the gym or sports?

The first few days to a week after the injection will be more focused on relative rest. This period is crucial to allow the PRP to work to its full effect. As a generalized rule, patients should avoid any activity that causes an increase in their pain. After the initial period of relative rest, it is essential to initiate a good rehabilitation program to focus on retraining the muscles and work on strength and range of motion. After discussing with your therapist and physician, you can choose the best time to return to your preferred gym routine or sport.

Will I need another injection?

Typically, repeat injections are not needed; however, this may vary based on location and the condition being treated. The effects of a single PRP can provide sufficient pain relief and functional improvement. For some patients, it is sometimes recommended to get a second "booster" injection at 3 months if they find that they are plateauing in their recovery and progress. During follow-up visits with your treating physician, there will be a discussion to either check in and continue, or there may need to be an adaptation of your plan.

How do I know if it's working?

With time, there should be a noticeable change in pain and function. Initially, the PRP injection may cause a temporary increase in pain. This is typically over the first week and is due to the activation of the inflammatory cascade. While you continue to progress further from the procedure and initiate a rehabilitation program, patients report dramatic reductions in pain with movements that previously caused them stress or harm.

How long will the PRP last?

The effects of PRP are variable from patient to patient. For some patients, the PRP can provide pain and functional relief for up to one year. For other patients, the results can last as long as three to five years. These effects are also dependent on focusing on strong physical therapy to help correct any biomechanical issues.

How long after the PRP can I start to take anti-inflammatory medications?

It is generally recommended to wait at least 4–6 weeks before resuming the anti-inflammatory medications and NSAIDs. The NSAIDs have antiplatelet properties that will diminish the effects of the PRP and may affect the recovery results.

Encouragement & Next Steps

The most important thing to remember is that this is a process. Please make sure to take the time to prioritize recovery after the injection. The healing process is gradual, and it's important to remember that. The other primary focus is getting into good rehabilitation to help retrain and strengthen those muscles to help the body further heal. Staying consistent in therapy will do wonders to help pay off results and improve the treatment outcomes. The next chapter will discuss further about good focuses for rehabilitation. It will discuss specific rehabilitation exercises and strengthening that may be incorporated to achieve the best results in recovery.

Bibliography

Arita, A., & Tobita, M. (2024). Adverse events related to platelet-rich plasma therapy and future issues to be resolved. *Regenerative Therapy*, *26*, 496–501. https://doi.org/10.1016/j.reth.2024.07.004

Block, J. E. (2010). Cold and compression in the management of musculoskeletal injuries and orthopedic operative procedures: A narrative review. *Open Access Journal of Sports Medicine*, *1*, 105–113. https://doi.org/10.2147/oajsm.s11102

Boswell, S. G., Cole, B. J., Sundman, E. A., Karas, V., & Fortier, L. A. (2012). Platelet-rich plasma: A milieu of bioactive factors. *Arthroscopy: The Journal of Arthroscopic & Related Surgery*, *28*(3), 429–439. https://doi.org/10.1016/j.arthro.2011.10.018

Brainard, B. M., Meredith, C. P., Callan, M. B., Budsberg, S. C., Shofer, F. S., Flaah, M., & Otto, C. M. (2007). Changes in platelet function, hemostasis, and prostaglandin expression after treatment with nonsteroidal anti-inflammatory drugs with various cyclooxygenase selectivities in dogs. *American Journal of Veterinary Research*, *68*(3), 251–257. https://doi.org/10.2460/ajvr.68.3.251

D'Souza, R. S., Her, Y. F., Hussain, N., Warner, N., Chon, J. Y., & Sayed, D. (2024). Evidence-based clinical practice guidelines on regenerative medicine treatment for chronic pain: A consensus report from a multispecialty working group. *Journal of Pain Research, 17*, 2951–3001. https://doi.org/10.2147/JPR.S480559

Hudgens, J. L., Sugg, K. B., Grekin, J. A., Gumucio, J. P., Bedi, A., & Mendias, C. L. (2016). Platelet-rich plasma activates proinflammatory signaling pathways and induces oxidative stress in tendon fibroblasts. *The American Journal of Sports Medicine, 44*(8), 1931–1940. https://doi.org/10.1177/0363546516637176

Jayaram, P., Kennedy, D. C., Yeh, P., & Dragoo, J. (2019). Chondrotoxic effects of local anesthetics on human knee articular cartilage: A systematic review. *PM&R, 11*(4), 379–400. https://doi.org/10.1002/pmrj.12007

Jayaram, P., Yeh, P., Patel, S. J., Mitchell, M., Shybut, T., & Navo, P. (2019). Effects of aspirin on growth factor release from freshly isolated leukocyte-rich platelet-rich plasma in healthy men: A prospective fixed-sequence controlled laboratory study. *The American Journal of Sports Medicine, 47*(5), 1223–1229. https://doi.org/10.1177/0363546519827294

Juneja, S. C., Schwarz, E. M., O'Keefe, R. J., & Awad, H. A. (2013). Cellular and molecular factors in flexor tendon repair and adhesions: A histological and gene expression analysis. *Connective Tissue Research, 54*(3), 218–226. https://doi.org/10.3109/03008207.2013.787418

Kaux, J. F., Forthomme, B., Namurois, M. H., Croisier, J. L., &

Crielaard, J. M. (2014). Description of a standardized rehabilitation program based on sub-maximal eccentric following a platelet-rich plasma infiltration for jumper's knee. *Muscles, Ligaments and Tendons Journal*, *4*(1), 85–89.

Khadavi, M., Pourcho, A., & Podesta, L. (2023). Protocols and techniques for orthobiologic procedures. *Physical Medicine and Rehabilitation Clinics of North America*, *34*(1), 105–115. https://doi.org/10.1016/j.pmr.2022.08.008

Knobloch, K., Grasemann, R., Spies, M., & Vogt, P. M. (2008). Midportion achilles tendon microcirculation after intermittent combined cryotherapy and compression compared with cryotherapy alone: A randomized trial. *The American Journal of Sports Medicine*, *36*(11), 2128–2138. https://doi.org/10.1177/0363546508319313

Kobayashi, E., Flückiger, L., Fujioka-Kobayashi, M., Sawada, K., Schaller, B., & Miron, R. J. (2016). Comparative release of growth factors from PRP, PRF, and advanced-PRF. *Clinical Oral Investigations*, *20*(9), 2353–2360. https://doi.org/10.1007/s00784-016-1719-1

Kumar, V., Abbas, A. K., & Aster, J. C. (2021). Tissue renewal and repair: Regeneration, healing, and fibrosis. In *Robbins and Cotran pathologic basis of disease* (10th ed., pp. 79–108). Elsevier.

Landén, N. X., Li, D., & Ståhle, M. (2016). Transition from

inflammation to proliferation: A critical step during wound healing. *Cellular and Molecular Life Sciences*, *73*(20), 3861–3885. https://doi.org/10.1007/s00018-016-2268-0

Levine, O. P., Kondapi, K., Tjong, V. K., & Gohal, C. (2024). Postinjection protocols following platelet-rich plasma administration for knee osteoarthritis: A systematic review. *PM&R*, *16*(9), 1023–1029. https://doi.org/10.1002/pmrj.13139

Lu, J., Li, H., Zhang, Z., Xu, R., Wang, J., & Jin, H. (2023). Platelet-rich plasma in the pathologic processes of tendinopathy: A review of basic science studies. *Frontiers in Bioengineering and Biotechnology*, *11*, Article 1187974. https://doi.org/10.3389/fbioe.2023.1187974

Mannava, S., Whitney, K. E., Kennedy, M. I., King, J. P., Evans, T. A., & LaPrade, R. F. (2019). The influence of naproxen on biological factors in leukocyte-rich platelet-rich plasma: A prospective comparative study. *Arthroscopy: The Journal of Arthroscopic & Related Surgery*, *35*(1), 201–210. https://doi.org/10.1016/j.arthro.2018.07.030

Mautner, K., Malanga, G., & Colberg, R. (2011). Optimization of ingredients, procedures and rehabilitation for platelet-rich plasma injections for chronic tendinopathy. *Pain Management*, *1*(6), 523–532. https://doi.org/10.2217/pmt.11.56

Middleton, K. K., Barro, V., Muller, B., Terada, S., & Fu, F. H. (2012). Evaluation of the effects of platelet-rich plasma (PRP) therapy involved in the healing of sports-related soft tissue injuries. *The Iowa Orthopaedic Journal, 32*, 150–163.

Park, A. L., Bailowitz, Z. P., Dejong, P. M., Shirazi, Z., Tsitsilianos, N., & von Richenbach, K. J. (2024). Postinjection protocols following platelet rich plasma injection for knee osteoarthritis: A systematic review of randomized controlled trials. *Journal of Cartilage & Joint Preservation*, *5*(1), Article 100201. https://doi.org/10.1016/j.jcjp.2023.100201

Pavlovic, V., Ciric, M., Jovanovic, V., & Stojanovic, P. (2016). Platelet-Rich Plasma: A short overview of certain bioactive components. *Open Medicine, 11*(1), 242–247. https://doi.org/10.1515/med-2016-0048

Reinke, J. M., & Sorg, H. (2012). Wound repair and regeneration. *European Surgical Research*, *49*(1), 35–43. https://doi.org/10.1159/000339613

Rubin, R., & Rand, M. L. (1994). Alcohol and platelet function. *Alcoholism: Clinical and Experimental Research, 18*(1), 105–110. https://doi.org/10.1111/j.1530-0277.1994.tb00888.x

Schippinger, G., Prüller, F., Divjak, M., Mahla, E., Fankhauser, F., Rehak, P., & Sprecher, C. (2015). Autologous platelet-rich plasma preparations: Influence of nonsteroidal anti-inflammatory drugs on platelet function. *Orthopaedic Journal of Sports Medicine, 3*(6), Article 2325967115588896. https://doi.org/10.1177/2325967115588896

Sharma, P., & Maffulli, N. (2006). Biology of tendon injury: Healing, modeling and remodeling. *Journal of Musculoskeletal and Neuronal Interactions, 6*(2), 181–190.

Sussman, W. I., Mautner, K., & Malanga, G. (2018). The role of rehabilitation after regenerative and orthobiologic procedures for the treatment of tendinopathy: A systematic review. *Regenerative Medicine, 13*(2), 249–263. https://doi.org/10.2217/rme-2017-0110

Sussman, W. I., Mautner, K., & Perone, A. (2022). Postprocedure considerations: Rehabilitation principles for interventional orthopedics and orthobiologics. In C. J. Williams, W. I. Sussman, & J. Pitts (Eds.), *Atlas of interventional orthopedics procedures* (pp. 599–611). Elsevier.

Townsend, C., Von Rickenbach, K. J., Bailowitz, Z., & Gellhorn, A. C. (2020). Post-procedure protocols following platelet-rich plasma injections for tendinopathy: A systematic review. *PM&R, 12*(9), 904–915. https://doi.org/10.1002/pmrj.12347

Voleti, P. B., Buckley, M. R., & Soslowsky, L. J. (2012). Tendon healing: Repair and regeneration. *Annual Review of Biomedical Engineering, 14*, 47–71. https://doi.org/10.1146/annurev-bioeng-071811-

150122

Zhang, Q. H., Das, K., Siddiqui, S., & Myers, A. K. (2000). Effects of acute, moderate ethanol consumption on human platelet aggregation in platelet-rich plasma and whole blood. *Alcoholism: Clinical and Experimental Research*, *24*(4), 528–534. https://doi.org/10.1111/j.1530-0277.2000.tb02021.x

CHAPTER 8

Post-PRP Rehabilitation

Authors: Joe Fiorelli & Kelly Terry

Introduction

This chapter begins by explaining why rehabilitation is essential for the success of platelet-rich plasma treatment. A well-structured, progressively loaded rehab program ensures the healing tissue adapts properly. This will reduce the risk of reinjury and support recovery. The following sections outline the key phases of exercise progression following PRP, detailing how and when to safely reintroduce load to support tissue healing and restore function. To optimize outcomes, the exercises and timeline for each rehabilitation phase are designed to align with the body's natural biological healing process.

During the **Acute Phase**, the primary goal is to restore range of motion and mobility. This prepares the joint and surrounding tissues for the loading phases that follow. In the

Early Strengthening Phase, the patient will initiate low-intensity loading to the involved structures while beginning to build stability in the surrounding musculature. The **Intermediate Strengthening Phase** emphasizes progressive overload to rebuild tissue capacity in the involved area, while continuing to build stability in the surrounding musculature.

For each of the initial three phases, there are five corresponding exercises. These exercises can be modified with regressions based on an individual's pain response and specific abilities. This guide utilizes the Pain Monitoring Model, which views total pain up to a 3 out of 10 as an acceptable 'safe' zone during activity. If pain spikes beyond these thresholds, it is recommended that the patient attempt one of the provided regressions. If pain remains elevated despite modifications, the individual should pause the exercises and consult a physician or doctor of physical therapy before continuing.

The **Advanced Functional Training Phase** aims to restore an individual to their pre-injury activity level. Unlike previous phases that focus on specific exercises, this phase is structured around the various stages of training principles. The effectiveness of this final phase hinges on selecting exercises that align with an individual's specific sport or functional goals. It is a guideline that may require critical thinking from the patient and/or consultation with a professional to determine the most suitable approach. This phase begins with Foundational Strength, progresses to Power Movements, then to Plyometrics, and finally to Sport-Specific Training.

Dr. Rothenberg's Shoulder PRP Progression Strategy

The following post-PRP rehabilitation exercises are based on Dr. Joshua Rothenberg's clinical experience treating patients following platelet-rich plasma (PRP) procedures over the past decade, in collaboration with Doctors of Physical Therapy who specialize in musculoskeletal rehabilitation. These recommendations serve as a general guideline; however, rehabilitation should always be individualized, and patients should consult their treating physician and rehabilitation team regarding the appropriate timing, progression, and specific exercises for their condition.

One of the most common challenges following platelet-rich plasma (PRP) treatment is determining the appropriate timing and progression of activity. While the biologic response begins immediately after the procedure, tissue remodeling and adaptation continue for weeks to months. For this reason, Dr. Rothenberg generally encourages patients to begin gentle, pain-limited range-of-motion exercises shortly after treatment, unless specific pathology or procedural considerations warrant additional protection. Early controlled motion may help maintain shoulder mobility, reduce stiffness, and promote appropriate tissue loading while respecting the healing process. More demanding strengthening exercises, recreational activities, sports, and occupational tasks are introduced in a gradual and structured manner.

Beginning at approximately two weeks after treatment, Dr. Rothenberg recommends resuming activity at roughly 25% of a patient's normal intensity and frequency (Figure 8.1). To guide progression, he uses a simple Green-Yellow-Red Zone system based on pain levels experienced during and after activity. The Green Zone represents mild discomfort (1–3 out of 10) that does not worsen during or after activity and is considered acceptable. The Yellow Zone represents moderate pain (4–6 out of 10), while the Red Zone represents significant pain (7–10 out of 10). Patients should only progress from 25% to 50%, then 75%, and ultimately 100% activity when they consistently remain in the Green Zone both during and after activity. Importantly, progression applies not only to exercise intensity but also to activity frequency.

If symptoms enter the Yellow or Red Zone, progression should be halted and activity should be reduced to the most recent level that consistently remained within the Green Zone. Once symptoms have returned to the Green Zone, progression may resume. This symptom-guided approach allows healing tissue to adapt gradually to increasing mechanical demands while minimizing the risk of symptom flare-ups and setbacks. The Green-Yellow-Red Zone progression model evolved through years of clinical experience, patient feedback, and continual refinement within Dr. Rothenberg's practice. Through extensive observation and trial-and-error across a wide range of shoulder pathologies, this strategy has become a practical framework for helping patients safely return to exercise, work, and sport following PRP treatment.

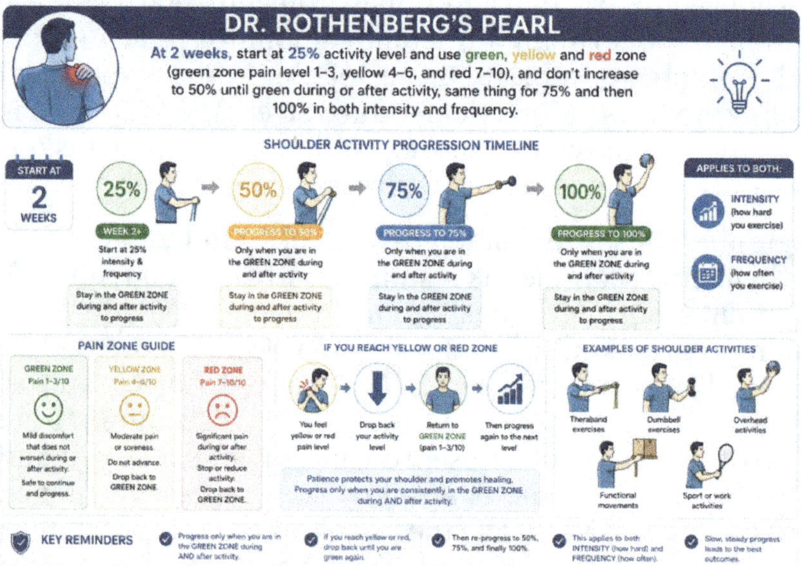

Figure 8.1 Dr. Rothenberg's Green Zone Rule for Returning to Activity After Shoulder PRP

This infographic outlines a structured return-to-activity progression following shoulder PRP treatment. Beginning at approximately 2 weeks post-procedure, patients start at 25% of their normal activity intensity and frequency and progress to 50%, 75%, and ultimately 100% only when they remain in the Green Zone (pain 1–3/10) during and after activity. If symptoms enter the Yellow Zone (pain 4–6/10) or Red Zone (pain 7–10/10), activity should be reduced, and patients should return to a Green Zone activity level before attempting further progression. This approach emphasizes gradual loading, symptom-guided rehabilitation, and avoidance of setbacks during the healing process.

Why Rehab is Crucial for PRP Success

Platelet-rich plasma therapy has become an increasingly popular intervention for managing chronic shoulder pain and soft tissue injuries. While promising in its biologic potential to accelerate healing, PRP is not a standalone solution. The regenerative process initiated by the injection must be supported through a thoughtfully designed and progressively loaded rehabilitation program.

Following a PRP injection, it's crucial to gradually increase forces on the involved structures through activity and exercise, rather than merely resting, to facilitate the healing process. This is because tissues will adapt based on the specific loads that are placed upon them. This adaptation is driven by mechanotransduction, where mechanical loads signal cells to align new collagen fibers along the direction of force to optimize function. Newly formed collagen and scar tissue will organize in a way that supports the direction of force the tissue is designed to use. For example, a tendon's physiological purpose is to withstand a tensile force. Adding a tensile force to a tendon during rehab will allow for new fibers to 'lay down' in a way that will optimize the tendon's ability to perform its function. If the tissue is underloaded, it will not adapt or strengthen effectively. On the other hand, if it is overloaded—whether too quickly or with excessive intensity—you risk tissue breakdown outpacing the rebuilding process. Both scenarios will increase the risk of reinjury and suboptimal healing.

To help safely implement these principles and ensure optimal tissue adaptation, a phased exercise program is essential. The following sections will provide a guide to a progressive loading approach that aligns with the healing timeline and functional demands of the involved structures.

Phase 1: Acute Phase

1. Supine Flexion AAROM with a Cane
    a. Description: *Lying on the back with knees bent and feet flat, a cane is held with both hands, palms facing down. The non-injured arm assists in lifting both arms overhead into shoulder flexion, keeping the elbows straight. After reaching a comfortable range, the arms are lowered back to the starting position.*
    b. Repetitions: 10-15
    c. Sets: 3
    d. Regression: *Limit the range of motion overhead*
    e. 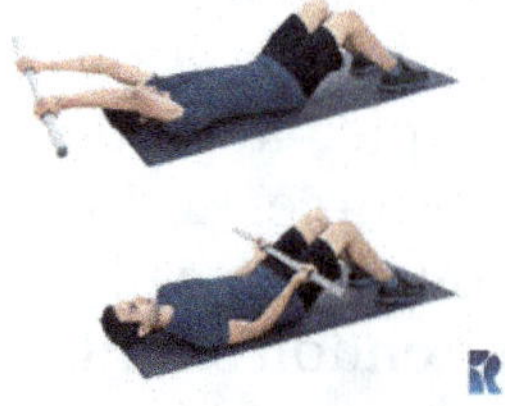

2. Supine Abduction AAROM with a cane

    a. Description: *Lying on the back with knees bent and feet flat, the palm of the affected arm faces upward. The unaffected arm assists in moving the affected arm outward into shoulder abduction, keeping both elbows straight. After reaching a comfortable range, the arms are lowered back to the starting position.*

    b. Repetitions: 10-15

    c. Sets: 3

    d. Regression: *Limit the range of motion*

    e.

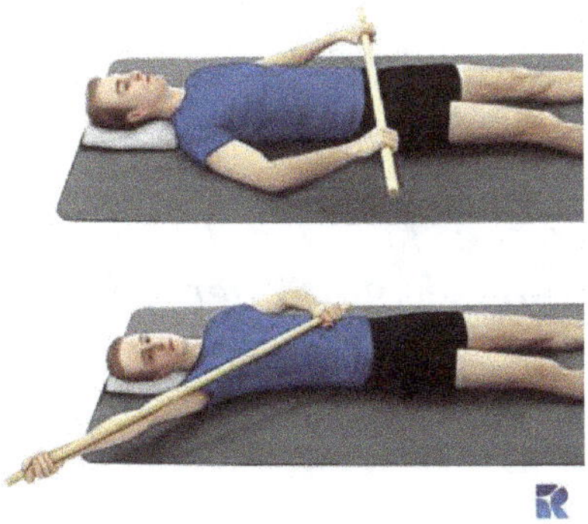

3. Scapular Retractions in Prone

    a. Description: *Lying face down, the shoulder blades are gently squeezed together, as if pinching a pencil between them. The contraction is held for 3 to 5 seconds, then relaxed. The shoulders should remain relaxed, without shrugging.*

b. Repetitions: 10-15

c. Sets: 3

d. Regression: *Perform in seated or standing position if unable to perform on stomach*

e.

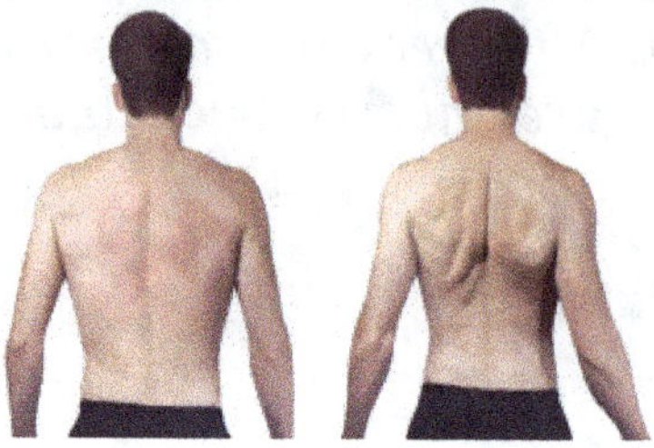

4. Isometric Internal Rotation

a. Description: *With the elbow bent at 90 degrees and tucked into the side, the palm is gently pressed into a wall or doorway without moving the shoulder. The contraction is held for 5 to 10 seconds, then relaxed.*

b. Repetitions: 10

c. Sets: 3

d. Regression: *Reduce the intensity or the duration of the inward press*

e.

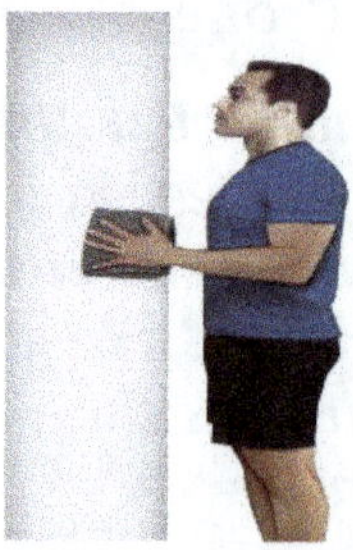

5. Isometric External Rotation

    a. Description: *With the elbow bent at 90 degrees and tucked into the side, the back of the hand is gently pressed into a wall or doorway without moving the shoulder. The contraction is held for 5 to 10 seconds, then relaxed.*

    b. Repetitions: 10

    c. Sets: 3

    d. Regression: *Reduce the intensity or the duration of the outward press*

    e.

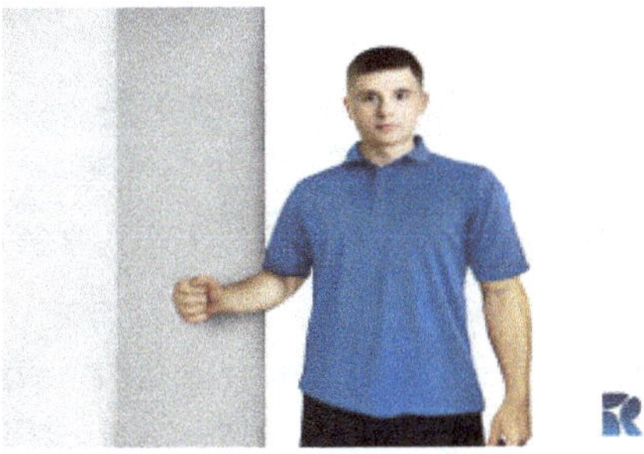

Phase 2: Early Strengthening Phase

1. Prone Y,T,I

    a. Description: *Lying face down with arms extended, the arms are lifted slightly off the ground in three positions: **I** – arms straight overhead, in line with the body. **Y** – arms angled out at 45 degrees. **T** – arms out to the sides at 90 degrees. In all positions, the elbows stay straight, thumbs point up, head remains down, and the shoulder blades engage without shrugging.*

b. Repetitions: 10 of each position

c. Sets: 3

d. Regression:

e.

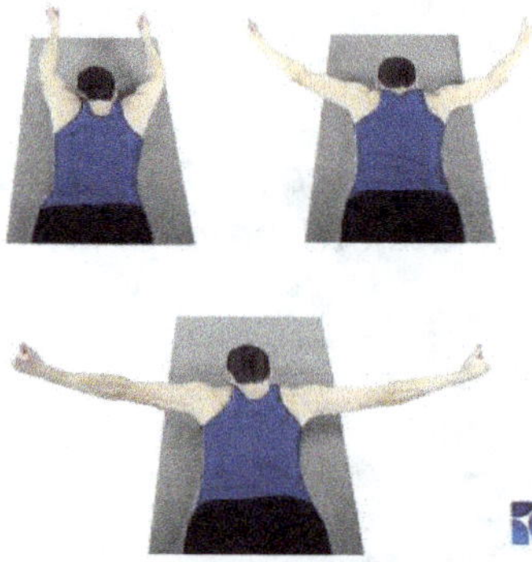

2. Side-lying Shoulder External Rotation with Scapular Retraction

    a. Description: *Lying on the side with the elbow bent to 90 degrees and tucked at the side, a light weight is held while the forearm rotates upward. At the same time, the shoulder blade is gently squeezed back and down. The elbow stays against the torso, wrist aligned with the forearm, and movement remains slow and controlled*

    b. Repetitions: 10-15

    c. Sets: 3

    d. Regression: *Reduce the weight and/or limit range of motion*

e.

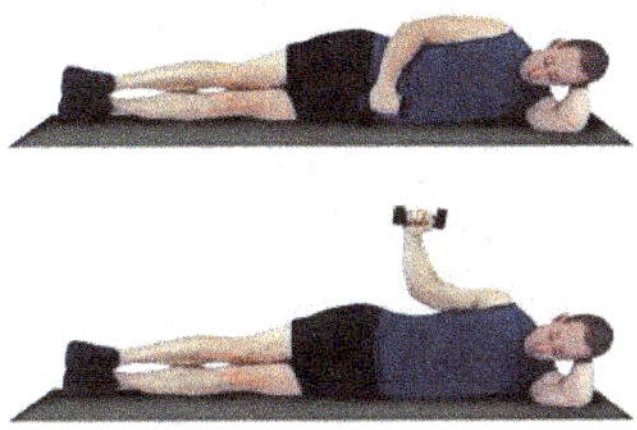

3. Resisted Shoulder External Rotation

    a. Description: *Standing with the elbow bent to 90 degrees and tucked at the side, a resistance band anchored at torso height is held. The forearm rotates outward against the band while keeping the elbow pinned and the shoulder relaxed. The movement is controlled, with a slow return to the starting position.*

    b. Repetitions: 10-15

    c. Sets: 3

    d. Regression: *Reduce level of resistance and/or limit range of motion*

    e.

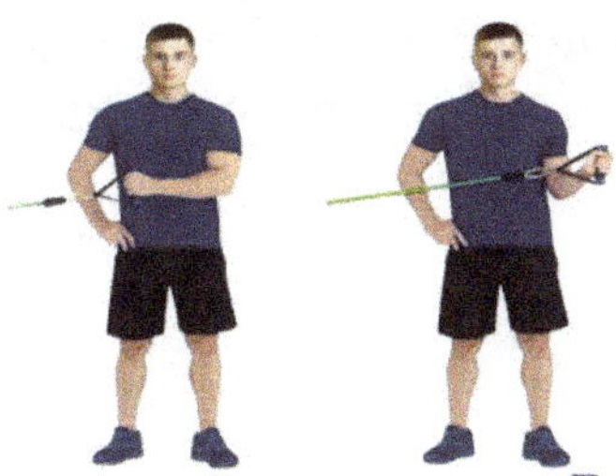

4. Resisted Shoulder Internal Rotation

    a. Description: *Standing with the elbow bent to 90 degrees and tucked at the side, a resistance band anchored at torso height is held. The forearm is pulled inward across the body against resistance, keeping the elbow close and shoulder relaxed. The motion is controlled throughout, especially on the return.*

    b. Repetitions: 10-15

    c. Sets: 3

    d. Regression: *Reduce level of resistance and/or limit range of motion*

    e.

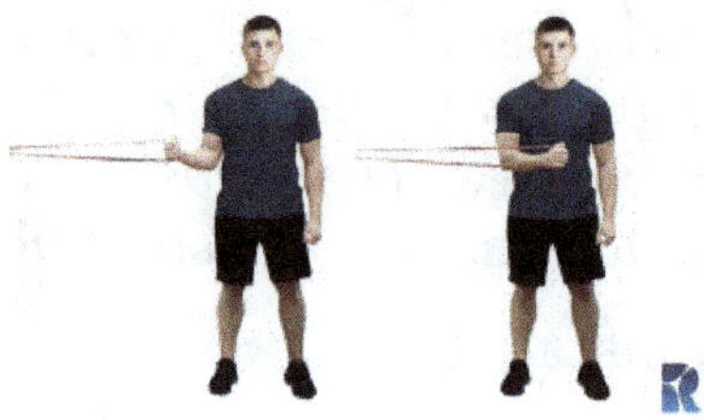

5. Standing DB raise in scapular plane

    a. Description: *Standing upright with light dumbbells at the sides and palms facing in, the arms are raised to shoulder height at a 45 degree angle from the front. Elbows stay straight, thumbs point up, and the motion is controlled without shrugging.*

    b. Repetitions: 10-15

    c. Sets: 3

    d. Regression: *Reduce weight and/or limit range of motion*

e.

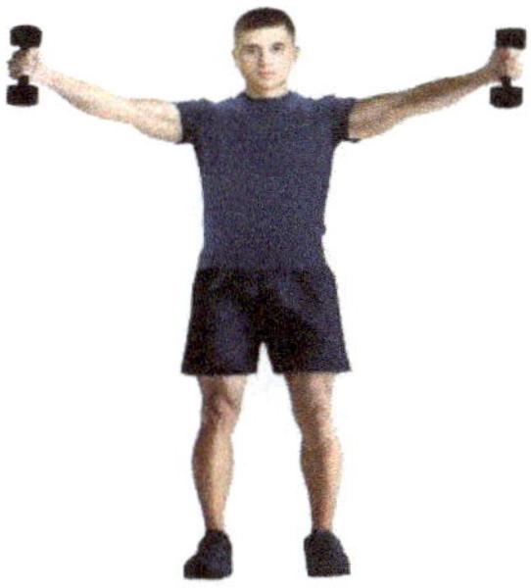

Phase 3: Intermediate Strengthening Phase

1. Resisted Seated Row

    a. Description: *Sitting with legs extended and a resistance band looped around the feet, the band is held with both hands and pulled toward the torso. The shoulder blades are squeezed together during the movement.*

    b. Repetitions: 8-12

    c. Sets: 3

    d. Regressions: *Reduce level of resistance and/or limit range of motion*

    e.

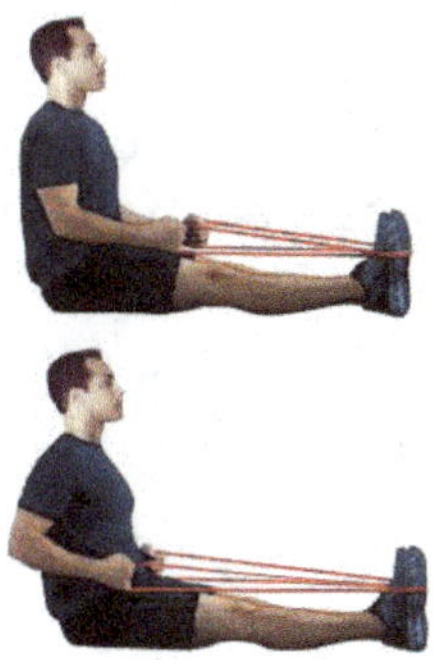

2. Resisted Lat Pulldown

    a. Description: *Seated or kneeling with a resistance band anchored overhead, the band is held with both hands, palms facing forward. It is pulled down toward the upper chest while squeezing the shoulder blades together, then slowly returned to the starting position with control.*

    b. Repetitions: 8-12

    c. Sets: 3

    d. Regressions: *Reduce level of resistance and/or limit range of motion*

    e. 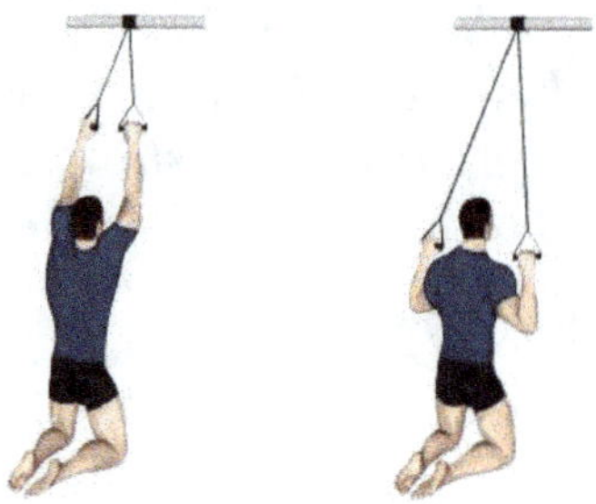

3. Dumbbell Floor Press

    a. Description: *Lying flat on the back with knees bent and a dumbbell in each hand, the elbows start at 90 degrees, resting on the floor. The dumbbells are pressed upward until the arms are fully extended, then slowly lowered back to the starting position.*

    b. Repetitions: 8-12

    c. Sets: 3

d. Regressions: *Reduce weight of dumbbells and/or limit range of motion.*

e.

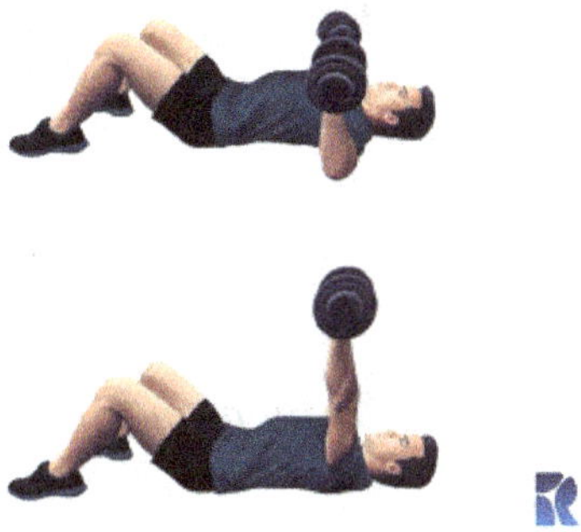

4. Forward Deltoid Raise with Dumbbells

   a. Description: *Holding weights at the sides, the arms are lifted straight forward to shoulder height, then slowly lowered with control.*

   b. Repetitions: 8-12

   c. Sets: 3

   d. Regressions: *Reduce weight and/or limit range of motion*

   e.

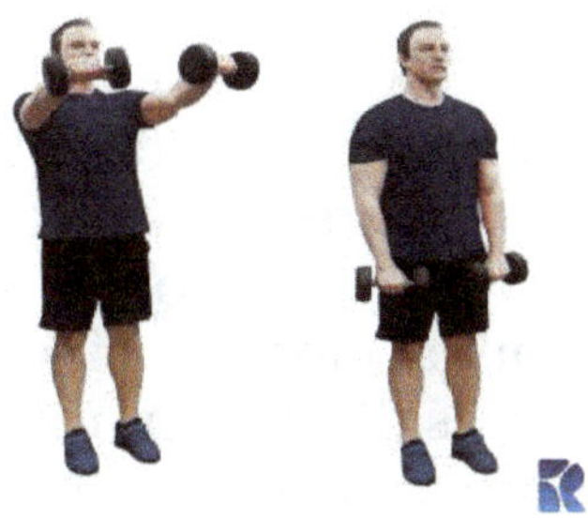

5. Side Deltoid Raise with Dumbbells
    a. Description: *Standing upright with a weight in each hand, the arms are lifted out to the sides to shoulder height, then slowly lowered back to the starting position.*
    b. Repetitions: 8-12
    c. Sets: 3
    d. Regressions: *Reduce weight and/or limit range of motion*
    e.

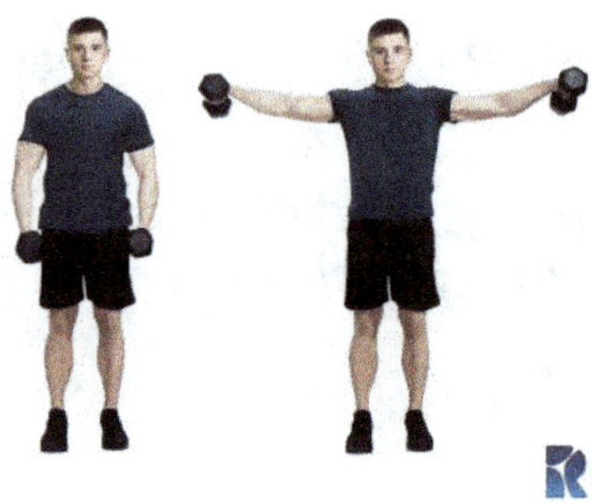

Phase 4: Advanced Functional Training Phase

Stage 1: Foundational Strength

This stage focuses on developing overall strength through multi-joint or compound movements, which engage multiple muscle groups simultaneously. The goal is to build a solid strength base that will support more specific training in later phases. For example, a tennis player aiming to improve their overhead serve might incorporate overhead dumbbell presses to build maximal force production throughout the upper extremity. This will lay the groundwork for more sport-specific movements in future stages.

- Example Movement: Dumbbell Overhead Press

  Description: *Standing upright with a dumbbell in each hand at shoulder height and palms facing forward, both dumbbells are pressed straight overhead until the arms are fully extended. Elbows remain slightly in front of the body throughout the movement.*

  Repetitions: 8-12

  Sets: 3

  Regressions: *Reduce weight and/or limit range of motion. Can also perform seated to increase external support*

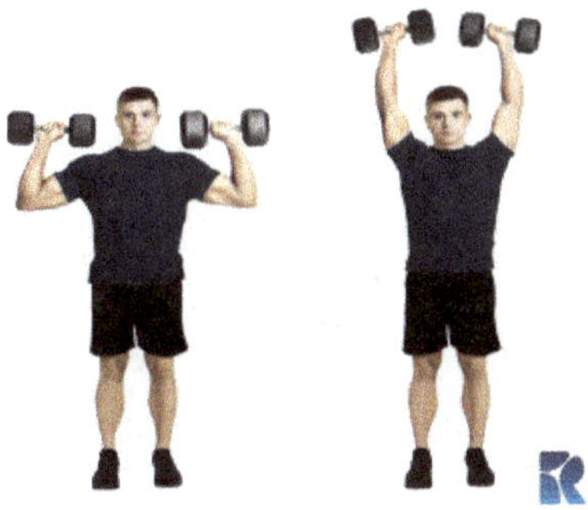

Stage 2: Power Movements

This stage emphasizes the ability to rapidly generate and absorb force through explosive, multi-joint movements. The goal is to transfer the foundational strength developed in earlier phases into powerful, sport-specific actions. For instance, a tennis player working to improve their overhead serve might perform medicine ball chop throws to simulate the quick, coordinated upper-body motion required during play.

- Example Movement: Medicine Ball Chop Throw

  Description: *Standing with feet shoulder-width apart and knees slightly bent, a medicine ball is held overhead and to one side. The athlete quickly rotates the trunk and drives the ball downward at an angle across the body, releasing it forcefully into the ground or wall. The movement mimics a chopping motion, engaging the core and shoulders.*

  Repetitions: 5-10

  Sets: 2-3

  Regression: *Reduce weight of ball, limit range of motion, and/or decrease speed of movement*

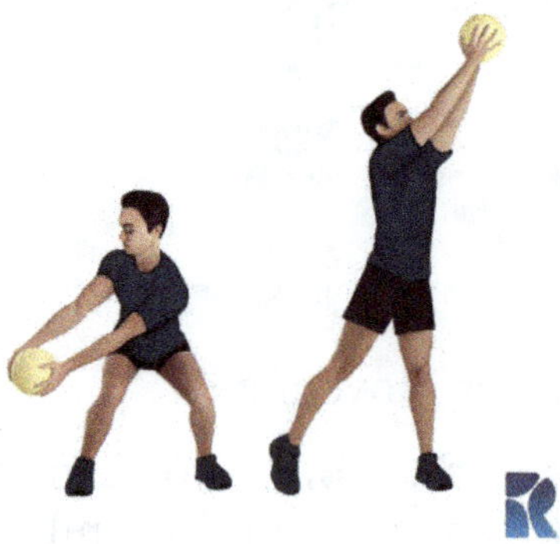

Stage 3: Plyometrics

Plyometric exercises train the body to move quickly and powerfully by utilizing a rapid stretch of the muscles immediately followed by a strong contraction. This takes advantage of the body's natural stretch reflex, similar to compressing and releasing a spring, which enhances the efficiency and explosiveness of muscular force production. Returning to the tennis serve example, a quick, explosive movement like a 90-90 wall ball throw helps reinforce power development in overhead patterns through the stretch-shortening cycle.

- Example Movement: 90/90 Wall Ball Throw

  Description: *Standing close to a wall in a throwing stance, the throwing arm is positioned at 90 degrees shoulder abduction and 90 degrees elbow flexion. The opposite leg is forward in a staggered stance. The shoulder externally rotates, then internally rotates to release the ball against the wall.*

  Repetitions: 10-15

  Sets: 3

  Regression: *Reduce weight of ball, limit range of motion, and/or decrease speed of movement*

  - 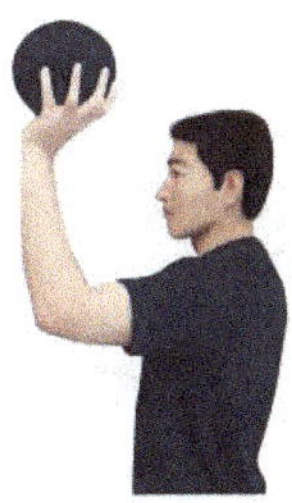

Stage 4: Sport-Specific Training

This stage marks the return to the actual movements the individual is aiming to perform in their sport or daily life. Training at this point closely replicates real-world or sport-specific activities. Returning to the tennis player example, this may involve practicing full overhead serves with a focus on refining technique to optimize performance.

- Example Movement: Shadow Tennis Serve with Racket

  Description: *A sport-specific drill reintroducing timing and mechanics of a tennis serve without impact. Gradually increase intensity and frequency.*

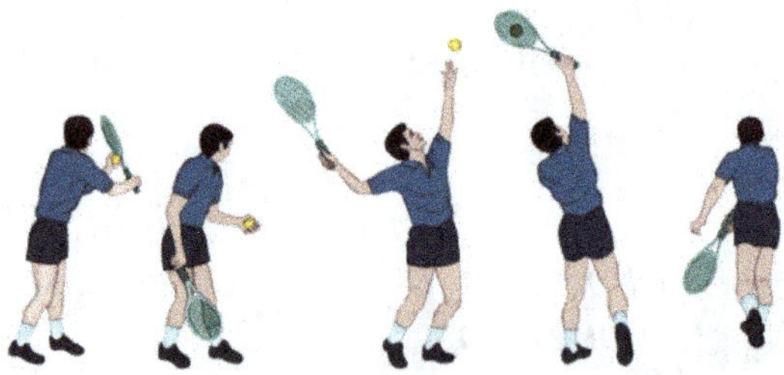

Bibliography

Khan, K. M., & Scott, A. (2009). Mechanotherapy: How physical therapists' prescription of exercise promotes tissue repair. *British Journal of Sports Medicine, 43*(4), 247–252. https://doi.org/10.1136/bjsm.2008.054239

Kawahara, T., Iida, S., Isoda, K., & Kim, S. (2024). Effects of platelet-rich plasma combined with exercise therapy for one year on knee osteoarthritis: Retrospective cohort study. *Journal of Orthopaedic Surgery and Research, 19*(1), Article 696. https://doi.org/10.1186/s13018-024-05186-w

Kisner, C., Colby, L. A., & Borstad, J. (2017). *Therapeutic exercise: Foundations and techniques* (7th ed.). F.A. Davis Company.

OpenAI. (2026). *ChatGPT* (May 2026 version) [Large language model]. https://chatgpt.com

Silbernagel, K. G., Thomeé, R., Eriksson, B. I., & Karlsson, J. (2007). Continued sports activity, using a pain-monitoring model, during rehabilitation in patients with Achilles tendinopathy: A randomized controlled study. *The American Journal of Sports Medicine, 35*(6), 897–906. https://doi.org/10.1177/0363546506298279

CHAPTER 9

Lifestyle & Nutrition for Optimization of Musculoskeletal Health

Author: Megan Ferderber

Introduction

Increasingly, we are learning that lifestyle habits are foundational to health, healing, and longevity. The musculoskeletal system forms the structural core of our bodies and is integral to our mobility and independence; therefore, leveraging lifestyle changes to optimize musculoskeletal health and healing is necessary for quality of life. Healthy lifestyle habits work synergistically with orthobiologic therapies and may aid treatment efficacy while also optimizing cell health, particularly the cells harvested for use in treatment and the cells that respond to each treatment. As the goal of orthobiologic therapy is to optimize the body's innate healing mechanisms, cellular health remains at the forefront of the musculoskeletal treatment algorithm. When we consider our cells used for orthobiologic treatments as our “medicine,” we want to have the best medicine possible, and therefore, we should regard our bodies as "pharmacies" and treat them as such. Lifestyle management should be regarded as important as, or even more important than, the orthobiologic procedure itself.

The practice of lifestyle medicine incorporates implementation of healthy habits following a system that includes six pillars: physical activity, sleep, stress reduction, nutrition, avoidance of risky substances, and social connectedness. Some of these pillars have greater roles in musculoskeletal health than others, but all contribute to overall improvement in cellular health. In this chapter, we review lifestyle medicine interventions and the evidence behind implementation to support bone, muscle, joint, and connective tissue health with the goal of assisting not only overall health and well-being but also improvement with orthobiologic treatments.

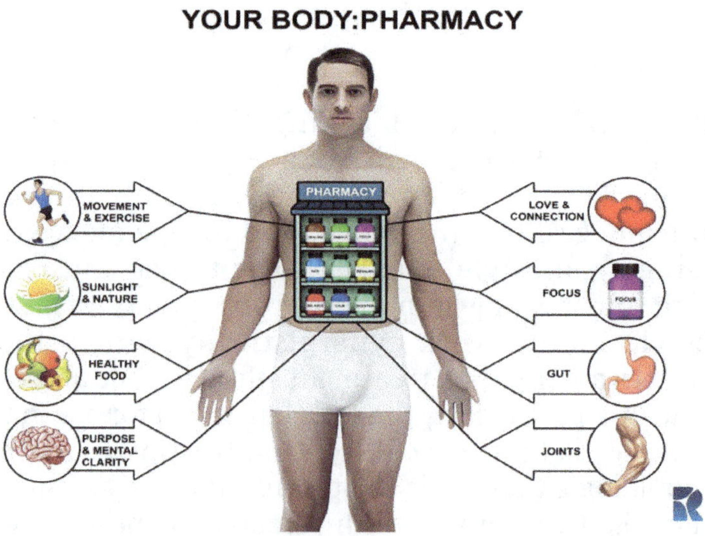

Figure 9.1 The Body as a Pharmacy: Foundations of Health and Recovery

This illustration highlights the concept that the body possesses powerful intrinsic healing mechanisms that can be influenced by daily lifestyle choices. Factors such as movement and exercise, nutrition, sunlight exposure, social connection, mental focus, purpose, gut health, and joint health act as important inputs that support overall wellness and tissue recovery. Optimizing these foundational elements may help create an environment that promotes resilience, recovery, and long-term musculoskeletal health.

Lifestyle Habits that Support Healing

Physical activity and exercise:

Exercise and physical activity have many known benefits to health, including decreasing overall mortality, cardiovascular disease, certain cancers, pain, and body fat. Systemic inflammation is also decreased with habitual exercise. Metabolic rate, bone density, strength, endurance, and sensitivity to insulin (which helps regulate glucose better) all increase with exercise. The gut microbiome, which is the balance of cells and healthy bacteria in the gastrointestinal tract, is kept healthy by exercise. In general, it is recommended by many medical organizations (American College of Sports Medicine, Centers for Disease Control, and American Heart Association) to complete 150 minutes of moderate-intensity aerobic activity per week, with strength training incorporated twice per week.

Exercise exerts an important effect on platelet amount and activity, which is an important consideration in PRP treatments. Acute exercise increases platelet circulation (released from the spleen). Twenty minutes of 70–85% maximum heart rate (MHR) exertion increased platelets, and 4 minutes of high-intensity exercise increased platelets and TGF-B; platelet function is increased with strenuous activity, but moderate activity decreases platelet activity in sedentary people.

Sleep

Sleep is imperative to the body's repair mechanisms, and therefore, quality sleep is necessary for musculoskeletal healing. In general, it is recommended that adults obtain 7–9 hours of sleep per night. Healthy sleep is linked to multiple advantages, including lower levels of the stress hormone cortisol, lower glucose levels, and better DNA repair. With poor sleep, there is an increased risk of cardiovascular disease, decreased testosterone and growth hormone, and immune system suppression.

Growth hormone is important in musculoskeletal health and tissue function, and is significantly impacted by sleep. The main roles of growth hormone are to stimulate growth, particularly in cartilage and bone, and to impact metabolism through increasing anabolic states of cells and protein synthesis. This process encourages tissue growth, repair, and recovery. Most growth hormone is released with the onset of deep sleep; quality sleep is necessary for appropriate growth hormone levels and release.

In regard to musculoskeletal health and musculoskeletal pain, there is emerging evidence that poor sleep in patients with osteoarthritis can contribute to hyperalgesia and faulty central pain modulation. This is likely due to the effects of sleep disruption on pain processing—poor sleep leads to abnormal pain processing and therefore impaired pain modulation.

We also know that conditions related to sleep, such as sleep apnea, are linked with abnormal platelet function due to increased platelet activation, which can additionally affect PRP treatments. Therefore, addressing sleep apnea and its risk factors may improve overall platelet function.

Avoidance of Risky Substances

Tobacco

If we regard our body as the source of our "medicine," we need to keep our medicine source free of contaminants. That's exactly the role that tobacco assumes in our body—it's an unhealthy contaminant, regarded by the CDC as a carcinogen and known to increase the risk of cancer, along with other chronic medical conditions. It impairs the immune system and contributes to slower wound healing. Tobacco use can lead to COPD, which can adversely affect platelet function. There is some evidence that smoking is associated with cartilage loss, while alcohol is associated with progression of disease and worsening of musculoskeletal conditions.

Cigarette smoking and nicotine can increase platelet aggregation and adhesion, which can adversely affect a PRP treatment. Therefore, it is advised to stop tobacco use or significantly cut back to help decrease this risk.

Alcohol

Alcohol is similarly regarded as a carcinogen by the CDC and is associated with cancer, stroke, and hypertension, among other chronic illnesses.

Alcohol can influence orthobiologics by directly damaging cells, resulting in altering cell function and disrupting cell signaling, which is imperative to the appropriate function of the cells necessary for healing. Even reducing alcohol in the short term can decrease surgical complications.

THC

Research on cannabis use and effects on cells utilized in orthobiologics is limited; there is some concern for adversely affecting bone healing and an increased risk of fracture.

Stress Management

More and more, unhealthy stress is recognized as a major contributor to chronic disease and poor overall body function. The key stress hormone is cortisol. Chronic stress and increased levels of cortisol, if unchecked, decrease the immune system function, increase inflammation, contribute to increased appetite and weight gain, and can increase clotting risk (affecting cells involved, including platelets), impair wound healing, telomere shortening, and insulin resistance. Strategies to manage stress can mitigate these effects. We know that stress can increase proinflammatory platelet activity, platelet aggregation, and proinflammatory state.

Meditation and mindfulness strategies can decrease stress and cortisol levels, with the goal of regulating unhealthy stress and therefore mitigating the adverse effects of cortisol on the body. These strategies can be set into motion with minimal time commitment, and can be as easy as dedicating five minutes daily to meditation, setting a mindfulness intention every morning prior to the start of the day, or following a structured program online or with a counselor or psychologist, depending on one's stress management needs

Social Connectedness

Social connectedness, while a separate aspect of lifestyle medicine from stress management, ties closely with all lifestyle changes, as social connectedness helps individuals adopt healthy lifestyle changes. Maintaining healthy relationships with family, friends, faith-based organizations, and work/school/volunteer colleagues permits positive emotions, the sense of meaning and accomplishment, and ultimately may promote longevity and mitigate disease risk.

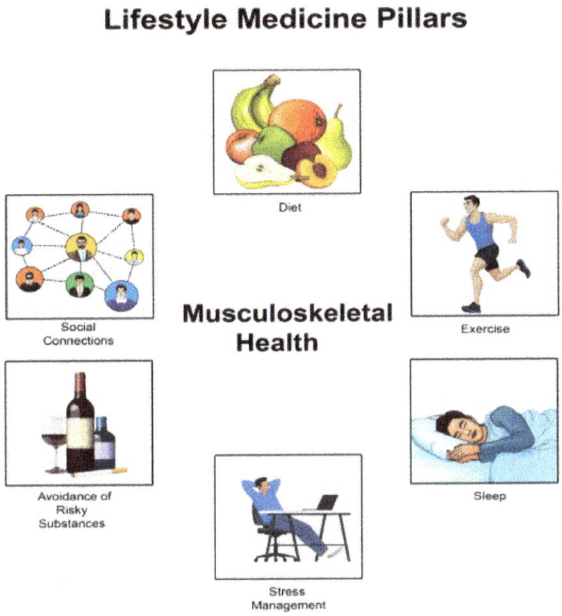

Figure 9.2 Lifestyle Medicine Pillars Supporting Musculoskeletal Health

This illustration highlights the six core pillars of lifestyle medicine that contribute to musculoskeletal health and overall well-being: nutrition, physical activity, restorative sleep, stress management, social connection, and avoidance of harmful substances. Together, these foundational lifestyle factors influence inflammation, recovery, physical function, tissue health, and long-term resilience, serving as important complements to medical and rehabilitative interventions.

Nutrition

The largest category of lifestyle intervention for health is nutrition. For musculoskeletal health, there are two different aspects of diet and nutrition that are important:

1. Indirect effects of diet (treatment of chronic conditions that contribute to poor musculoskeletal health, i.e., obesity, diabetes, etc.)
2. Direct effects of diet (anti-inflammatory effects that are good for cell function and cell health; tissue repair)

Indirect Effects of Diet

Nutrition takes a front row seat in the prevention of many chronic conditions, such as obesity, metabolic syndrome, hyperlipidemia/dyslipidemia, hypertension, diabetes, etc. Nutrition even has a role in cancer, with poor nutrition and diets high in ultra-processed foods linked to certain types of gastrointestinal cancers, which are currently on the rise in younger populations. Appropriate nutrition is also known to treat and reverse chronic diseases, making it a powerhouse lifestyle intervention for many conditions and the many people afflicted.

Direct Effects of Diet

Inflammation Modulation

It is important to understand the two types of inflammation and the various roles they play in musculoskeletal healing and repair: acute and chronic inflammation.

Acute inflammation is the quick response to tissue injury involving cells with roles and responsibilities to initiate tissue repair. This is an important process necessary for tissue healing and regeneration.

Chronic inflammation, on the other hand, occurs when the acute inflammatory phase fails to resolve the issue or injury, leading to continued production of inflammatory molecules and other cellular processes that increase oxidative stress and actually impair healing.

Diets like the Mediterranean diet and the anti-inflammatory diet ideally incorporate foods and food groups daily that are known to minimize inflammation and promote anti-inflammatory and antioxidant effects on the body. Both diets are characterized by high levels of intake of vegetables and fruits, in addition to nuts, legumes, grains, and fatty fish, and limiting processed foods and meats while minimizing added sugars. The anti-inflammatory diet also incorporates antioxidant-rich foods like berries, spices like turmeric, and herbs. The anti-inflammatory and anti-oxidant effects promote musculoskeletal health and healing, and can work with your body's innate healing ability when proceeding with orthobiologic treatments. Figure 9.3 demonstrates recommended anti-inflammatory foods that serve as a foundation to healthy daily nutrition that can support musculoskeletal health and orthobiologic treatment.

Achieving a balance of omega-3 and omega-6 fatty acids can support musculoskeletal healing through limiting pro-inflammatory signaling and promoting anti-inflammatory pathways. Both types of fatty acids are considered polyunsaturated, but differ in their function. An excess in consumption of omega-6 fatty acids can exacerbate chronic inflammation and lead to impaired healing and cartilage degeneration, whereas omega-3 fatty acids lead to anti-inflammatory pathways and reduce oxidative stress, thus supporting musculoskeletal healing. Maintaining a nutritional intake ratio of omega-6/omega-3 fatty acids between 1:1 and 4:1 has been shown to have advantageous effects on cartilage. Common sources of both omega-3 and omega-6 fatty acids are listed below.

Table 9.1 Common Sources of Omega-3 and Omega-6 Fatty Acids

Sources of Omega-3 Fatty Acids	Sources of Omega-6 Fatty Acids
Salmon	Tofu
Mackerel	Eggs
Sardines	Peanut butter
Flaxseeds	Sunflower seeds
Chia seeds	Sesame seeds
Walnuts	Vegetable oils

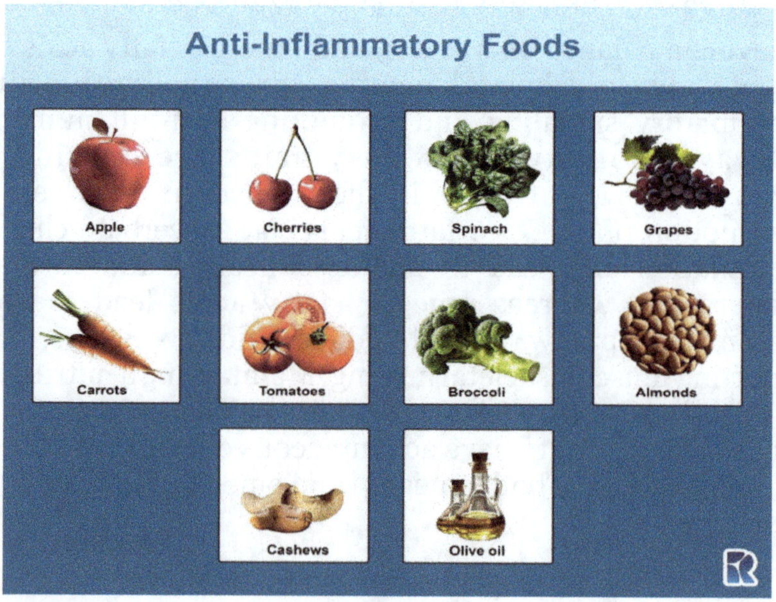

Figure 9.3 Dietary Sources of Nutrients Associated with Anti-Inflammatory Effects

This illustration highlights several nutrient-dense foods commonly associated with anti-inflammatory dietary habits, including fruits, vegetables, nuts, and healthy fats. These foods contain vitamins, minerals, antioxidants, polyphenols, and other bioactive compounds that may help support overall health, regulate inflammatory processes, and promote recovery. Incorporating a variety of whole foods into the diet may complement musculoskeletal health and wellness efforts.

Tissue Repair

Protein

The role of diet in musculoskeletal tissue repair is quite complex; however, one of the main building blocks is protein. Protein is integral in collagen synthesis as it supplies the necessary amino acids. Recall that collagen is the most abundant protein in our bodies and provides structure to our musculoskeletal system, as it is the main component of bones (type I collagen), cartilage (type II collagen), and tendons and ligaments (mostly type 1 collagen).

Recommendations for ideal amounts of daily protein vary; however, the general guideline for a healthy adult is to consume a minimum of 0.8–1.0 g/kg body weight daily, with recommendations increasing to 1.2–2.0 g/kg body weight daily for athletes, and sometimes higher (2.0–2.5 g/kg daily) in conditions where significant healing and tissue turnover are necessary.

While bodies can create the amino acids needed for collagen synthesis, the most important of which is glycine, dietary sources are often needed in high-demand states such as wound healing, growth, or tissue repair. Dietary protein can be increased through both animal-based and plant-based sources, with examples below including approximate amounts of protein per listed serving:

Table 9.2 Common Animal- and Plant-Based Protein Sources and Their Approximate Protein Content

Animal-based	Protein (g)	Plant-based	Protein (g)
Chicken breast (3–4 oz)	25–35 g	Tofu (3.5 oz)	17 g
Turkey breast (3 oz)	24 g	Edamame (1 cup)	18.5 g
Beef sirloin (3 oz)	22–26 g	Lentils (1/2 cup)	12 g
Tuna (5 oz)	30–35 g	Chickpeas (1/2 cup)	7 g
Salmon (3–4 oz)	22–25 g	Black beans (1/2 cup)	8 g
Eggs (1 large egg)	6–7 g	Almonds (1 oz)	6 g
Greek yogurt (6–7 oz)	15–20 g	Pumpkin seeds (1 oz)	7–10 g
Cow's milk (8 oz)	8 g	Hemp seeds (3 tbsp)	10 g
Cottage cheese (1/2 cup)	12 g	Chia seeds (1 oz)	5 g

Collagen supplements have become popular adjuncts to a healthy diet, with some evidence demonstrating that hydrolyzed collagen supplements, along with exercise, can improve collagen synthesis in the body, especially at a dose of 30 g/day. There is currently no research demonstrating that collagen supplementation is superior to adequate dietary intake of protein, but there is evidence that collagen supplements are as effective as dietary protein in supporting collagen synthesis.

Vitamins and Minerals

Tendon and ligament repair processes are facilitated by adequate amounts of key vitamins and minerals, such as vitamin C, zinc, copper, vitamin D, and magnesium. While these elements are commonly encountered in a healthy diet, supplementation may be beneficial in states where tissue turnover and healing occur.

Vitamin C is an essential element for synthesizing collagen and stabilizing collagen fibers, as it acts as a cofactor (helps in the functioning of enzymes needed to make collagen). Vitamin C also decreases oxidative stress and accelerates tendon healing. In particular, following injury, Vitamin C supplementation improves function and tendon tissue organization. The optimal dose of vitamin C as a supplement is unknown at this time, but as it is a water-soluble vitamin and is excreted through urine if in high amounts, there is little concern for taking too much.

Like Vitamin C, zinc is also a cofactor and is important in remodeling the extracellular matrix and assisting cell proliferation and immune function. Zinc plays a role in tissue repair, and deficiencies in zinc lead to poor and delayed wound healing. There is little evidence for zinc supplementation specifically for the repair of musculoskeletal structures, but its role in wound healing is well known.

Copper assists an enzyme responsible for cross-linking and stabilizing collagen and the extracellular matrix, therefore strengthening musculoskeletal tissue. Copper can increase biomechanical strength and is integral in tissue repair in this regard.

Vitamin D and magnesium work together, as magnesium is necessary for the activation of vitamin D, and vitamin D assists in the bodily absorption of magnesium. Adequate amounts of both are necessary for musculoskeletal healing and tissue repair, as well as optimizing bone health and decreasing inflammation.

Table 9.3 Key Micronutrients Involved in Musculoskeletal Tissue Repair and Healing

Micronutrient	Role in tissue repair/healing:	Recommended daily amount*:
Vitamin C	Collagen synthesis and antioxidant	90 mg—Men 75 mg—Women
Zinc	Remodeling of the extracellular matrix and tissue repair/wound healing	11 mg—Men (age 19 and older) 8 mg—Women (age 19 and older)
Copper	Stabilization of collagen and extracellular matrix; strengthens musculoskeletal tissue	900 mg—19 years and older
Vitamin D	Musculoskeletal healing and repair; works with magnesium	400 IU—up to age 12 mo 600 IU—ages 1–70 years 800 IU—over 70 years
Magnesium	Musculoskeletal healing and repair; works with Vitamin D	400–420 mg—Men 310–320 mg—Women

*amounts vary based on chronic disease states, ages, or other specific conditions (e.g. pregnancy).

Special Considerations: Effects of Diet on Cell Products

Specifically, when considering orthobiologic treatments in the setting of nutrition, high-fat and high-calorie diets can impede the function of many cells utilized. Additionally, high-fat and high-cholesterol meals can impact the quality of cells harvested for treatment through processing and preparation for use in injections (e.g., a fatty meal prior to having blood drawn for PRP may result in a poor blood sample and too much fat in the product).

How Diet Can Play a Role in Osteoarthritis

Diet has a particularly important role in osteoarthritis, given the benefits of diet in treating and decreasing the risk of obesity and metabolic syndrome. Obesity is defined as a BMI at or greater than 30 kg/m^2, whereas metabolic syndrome is defined by an individual meeting a minimum of three risk factors that increase the risk of type 2 diabetes and cardiovascular disease.

The risk factors for metabolic syndrome are the following:

1. Increased waist circumference–in the United States, these cut-off values are greater than 102 cm in men and greater than 88 cm in women.
2. Elevated fasting glucose level–this is a fasting glucose level greater than or equal to 100 mg/dL.
3. Elevated blood pressure–having blood pressure at or greater than 130/85 mm Hg.
4. Elevated triglycerides–triglycerides greater than or equal to 150 mg/dL.
5. Reduced HDL (good) cholesterol–men with HDL less than mg/dL and women with HDL less than 50 mg/dL are considered to have low HDL.

While not a specific criterion for metabolic syndrome, individuals with an unhealthy BMI often run the risk of meeting the criteria for metabolic syndrome (ex. increased waist circumference, in addition to lab values demonstrating poor metabolic function).

With obesity and metabolic syndrome, osteoarthritis can be affected by two different pathways:

Pathway A—Mechanical load on joints: excess weight can place an increased burden and pressure on joints, particularly weight-bearing joints, which can then lead to joint pain, wear down cartilage, and worsen osteoarthritis.

- Research has shown that one pound of weight loss can equal a 4-fold reduction in load on the knee per step.
- Weight loss improves the quality and quantity of cartilage in the knee.

The role of diet and nutrition in pathway A is to aid in maintaining a healthy weight, fight obesity, and decrease mechanical load on joints.

Pathway B—Metabolic effects on joints: a combination of metabolic processes that inhibit or retard the body's repair processes. These stem from poor health status, such as having abnormal lipid levels in the body (dyslipidemia), having increased levels of serum glucose (insulin resistance), and an imbalance of the gut bacteria (microbiota dysbiosis). The figure below demonstrates the complex metabolic pathways that lead to joint degeneration: microbiota dysbiosis, bad cholesterol (LDL), elevated glucose, and increases in factors called adipokines released from adipose/fatty tissue lead to low-grade inflammation and oxidative stress on cells, which alter the function of cells within joints and lead to joint degradation and degeneration (Figure 9.4).

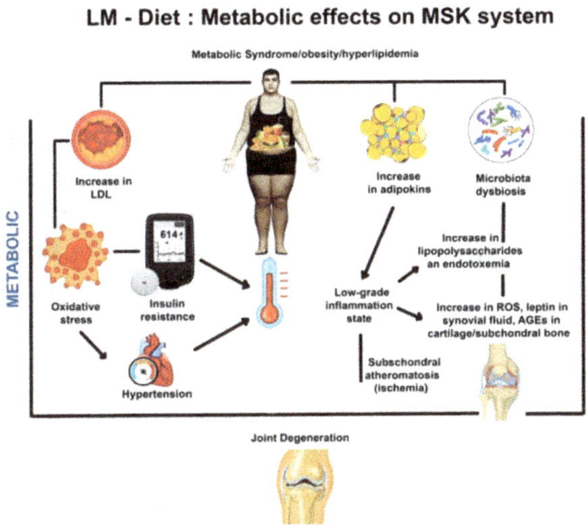

Figure 9.4 The Impact of Diet and Metabolic Health on Musculoskeletal Disease

This illustration demonstrates how poor dietary habits and metabolic dysfunction may contribute to musculoskeletal disease through both metabolic and mechanical pathways. Obesity, insulin resistance, dyslipidemia, oxidative stress, hypertension, altered adipokine signaling, and gut microbiome dysbiosis can promote chronic low-grade inflammation and increase inflammatory mediators within musculoskeletal tissues. These processes may adversely affect cartilage, synovium, subchondral bone, and other joint structures, ultimately contributing to pain, degeneration, and osteoarthritis progression. Additionally, excess body weight increases mechanical loading across joints, further accelerating tissue breakdown and functional decline.

The role of diet and nutrition in pathway B is to maintain metabolic homeostasis in the body, as diet has been shown to aid in balancing gut bacteria, optimizing cholesterol, minimizing insulin resistance, and decreasing inflammation and oxidative stress.

In considering the significant impact of nutrition on both pathways with joint degeneration, when proceeding with orthobiologic treatments, such as PRP, it becomes important to prioritize the need to optimize the body's metabolic influence on musculoskeletal health and healing, and decrease mechanical load on weight-bearing joints through nutrition.

Key Takeaways

- A healthy body and lifestyle can facilitate musculoskeletal health and healing and support orthobiologic therapies.
- Lifestyle medicine pillars, such as exercise, nutrition, sleep, stress management, social connectedness, and avoidance of risky substances, promote overall health and play a role in musculoskeletal healing.
- There is a role for certain supplements in aiding the healing environment of the body, and therefore, it is recommended to optimize these in dietary intake or supplementation to improve overall health.
- Foods rich in anti-inflammatory and antioxidant properties support decreasing overall inflammation and oxidative stress and therefore can support musculoskeletal and bodily health.

Bibliography

Aaboe, J., Bliddal, H., Messier, S. P., Alkjær, T., & Henriksen, M. (2011). Effects of an intensive weight loss program on knee joint loading in obese adults with knee osteoarthritis. *Osteoarthritis and Cartilage*, *19*(7), 822–828. https://doi.org/10.1016/j.joca.2011.03.006

Anz, A. W., Parsa, R. S., Romero-Creel, M. F., Smith, M. J., & Sherman, S. L. (2019). Exercise-mobilized platelet-rich plasma: Short-term exercise increases stem cell and platelet concentrations in platelet-rich plasma. *Arthroscopy: The Journal of Arthroscopic & Related Surgery*, *35*(1), 192–200. https://doi.org/10.1016/j.arthro.2018.06.043

Baria, M. R., Miller, M. M., Borchers, J., McShane, K., Kim, J., & Magnussen, R. (2020). High intensity interval exercise increases platelet and transforming growth factor-β yield in platelet-rich plasma. *PM&R*, *12*(12), 1244–1250. https://doi.org/10.1002/pmrj.12368

Chapman, L., Ren, T., Solka, J., & Taylor, S. (2023). Reducing alcohol use before and after surgery: Qualitative study of two treatment approaches. *JMIR Perioperative Medicine*, *6*, Article e42532. https://doi.org/10.2196/42532

Clayton, J. S. (2023). *Foundations of lifestyle medicine board review manual* (4th ed.). American College of Lifestyle Medicine.

de Paz-Lugo, P., Lupiáñez, J. A., & Meléndez-Hevia, E. (2018). High glycine concentration increases collagen synthesis by articular chondrocytes in vitro: Acute glycine deficiency could be an important cause of osteoarthritis. *Amino Acids*, *50*(10), 1357–1365. https://doi.org/10.1007/s00726-018-2611-x

Dominguez, L. J., Veronese, N., Ragusa, F. S., Solis-Navarro,

L., Ciriminna, G., & Barbagallo, M. (2025). The importance of vitamin D and magnesium in athletes. *Nutrients*, *17*(10), Article 1655. https://doi.org/10.3390/nu17101655

Eliasen, M., Grønkjær, M., Skov-Ettrup, L. S., Mikkelsen, S. S., Becker, U., Flensborg-Madsen, T., & Grønbæk, M. (2013). Preoperative alcohol consumption and postoperative complications: A systematic review and meta-analysis. *Annals of Surgery*, *258*(6), 930–942. https://doi.org/10.1097/SLA.0b013e3182988d59

Furman, D., Campisi, J., Verdin, E., Carrera-Bastos, P., Targ, S., Franceschi, C., Lopez-Otin, C., Melov, S., Newgard, C. B., Cordain, L., Schulz, L. O., Chan, S. B., Paolo, G., & Slavich, G. M. (2019). Chronic inflammation in the etiology of disease across the life span. *Nature Medicine*, *25*(12), 1822–1832. https://doi.org/10.1038/s41591-019-0675-0

Harasymowicz, N. S., Dicks, A., Wu, C. L., & Guilak, F. (2019). Physiologic and pathologic effects of dietary free fatty acids on cells of the joint. *Annals of the New York Academy of Sciences*, *1440*(1), 36–53. https://doi.org/10.1111/nyas.13999

Heath, D. M., Koslosky, E. J., Bartush, K. C., & Hogue, G. D. (2022). Marijuana in orthopaedics: Effects on bone health, wound-healing, surgical complications, and pain management. *JBJS Reviews*, *10*(2), Article e21.00184. https://doi.org/10.2106/JBJS.RVW.21.00184

Heymsfield, S. B., & Shapses, S. A. (2024). Guidance on energy and macronutrients across the life span. *New England Journal of Medicine*, *390*(14), 1299–1310. https://doi.org/10.1056/NEJMra2214275

Jiménez-Muro, M., Soriano-Romaní L., Mora, G., Ricciardelli, D., & Nieto, J. A. (2023). The microbiota-metabolic syndrome axis as a promoter of metabolic osteoarthritis. *Life Sciences*, *329*, Article 121944. https://doi.org/10.1016/j.lfs.2023.121944

Khatri, M., Naughton, R. J., Clifford, T., Harper, L. D., & Corr, L. (2021). The effects of collagen peptide supplementation on body composition, collagen synthesis, and recovery from joint injury and exercise: A systematic review. *Amino Acids*, *53*(10), 1493–1506. https://doi.org/10.1007/s00726-021-03072-x

Kheyruri, F., Sarrafzadeh, J., Hosseini, A. F., Abiri, B., & Vafa, M. (2021). Randomized study of the effects of vitamin D and magnesium co-supplementation on muscle strength and function, body composition, and inflammation in vitamin D-deficient middle-aged women. *Biological Trace Element Research*, *199*(7), 2523–2534. https://doi.org/10.1007/s12011-020-02387-2

Kontos, A., Willoughby, S., Lushington, K., Martin, J., Scott, H., & Catcheside, P. (2020). Increased platelet aggregation in children and adolescents with sleep-disordered breathing. *American Journal of Respiratory and Critical Care Medicine*, *202*(11), 1560–1566. https://doi.org/10.1164/rccm.201911-2229OC

Lee, J., Tang, J. C. Y., Dutton, J., Dunn, R., Fraser, W. D., & Johnston, R. (2024). The collagen synthesis response to an acute bout of resistance exercise is greater when ingesting 30 g hydrolyzed collagen compared with 15 g and 0 g in resistance-trained young men. *The Journal of Nutrition*, *154*(7), 2076–2086. https://doi.org/10.1016/j.tjnut.2023.10.030

Lippi, G., Mattiuzzi, C., & Franchini, M. (2015). Sleep apnea and venous thromboembolism: A systematic review. *Thrombosis and Haemostasis*, *114*(5), 958–963.

https://doi.org/10.1160/TH15-03-0188

Mao, H., Lu, G., Zheng, L., & Wang, Y. (2025). The research progress and potential applications of omega-3 fatty acids in orthopedics: A narrative review. *British Journal of Nutrition*. Advance online publication. https://doi.org/10.1017/S0007114525103875

Messier, S. P., Gutekunst, D. J., Davis, C., & DeVita, P. (2005). Weight loss reduces knee-joint loads in overweight and obese older adults with knee osteoarthritis. *Arthritis & Rheumatism*, *52*(7), 2026–2032. https://doi.org/10.1002/art.21139

Milewska, M., Burdzińska, A., Zielniok, K., Dybowska, M., Zarychta, K., & Kawiak, J. (2020). Copper does not induce tenogenic differentiation but promotes migration and increases lysyl oxidase activity in adipose-derived mesenchymal stromal cells. *Stem Cells International*, *2020*, Article 9123281. https://doi.org/10.1155/2020/9123281

Noriega-González, D. C., Drobnic, F., Caballero-García, A., Roche, E., Perez-Valdecantos, D., & Córdova, A. (2022). Effect of vitamin C on tendinopathy recovery: A scoping review. *Nutrients*, *14*(13), Article 2663. https://doi.org/10.3390/nu14132663

Rogerson, O., Wilding, S., Prudenzi, A., & O'Connor, D. B. (2024). Effectiveness of stress management interventions to change cortisol levels: A systematic review and meta-analysis. *Psychoneuroendocrinology*, *159*, Article 106415. https://doi.org/10.1016/j.psyneuen.2023.106415

Saeg, F., Orazi, R., Bowers, G. M., & Janis, J. E. (2021). Evidence-based nutritional interventions in wound care. *Plastic and Reconstructive Surgery*, *148*(1), 226–238. https://doi.org/10.1097/PRS.0000000000008061

Smith, M. T., Quartana, P. J., Okonkwo, R. M., & Nasir, A. (2009). Mechanisms by which sleep disturbance contributes to osteoarthritis pain: A conceptual model. *Current Pain and Headache Reports*, *13*(6), 447–454. https://doi.org/10.1007/s11916-009-0073-2

Soliman, A. M., & Barreda, D. R. (2022). Acute inflammation in tissue healing. *International Journal of Molecular Sciences*, *24*(1), Article 641. https://doi.org/10.3390/ijms24010641

Tack, C., Shorthouse, F., & Kass, L. (2018). The physiological mechanisms of effect of vitamins and amino acids on tendon and muscle healing: A systematic review. *International Journal of Sport Nutrition and Exercise Metabolism*, *28*(3), 294–311. https://doi.org/10.1123/ijsnem.2017-0267

Van Cauter, E., Kerkhofs, M., Caufriez, A., Van Onderbergen, A., Thorner, M. O., & Copinschi, G. (1992). A quantitative estimation of growth hormone secretion in normal man: Reproducibility and relation to sleep and time of day. *The Journal of Clinical Endocrinology & Metabolism*, *74*(6), 1441–1450. https://doi.org/10.1210/jcem.74.6.1592892

Wang, J. S., Jen, C. J., Kung, H. C., Lin, L. J., Hsiue, T. R., & Chen, H. I. (1994). Different effects of strenuous exercise and moderate exercise on platelet function in men. *Circulation*, *90*(6), 2877–2885. https://doi.org/10.1161/01.cir.90.6.2877

Wieczorek, M., Gwinnutt, J. M., Ransay-Colle, M., Balanescu, A., Barros, R., Radu, R. I., & Euller-Ziegler, L. (2022). Smoking, alcohol consumption and disease-specific outcomes in rheumatic and musculoskeletal diseases (RMDs): Systematic reviews informing the 2021 EULAR recommendations for lifestyle improvements in people with RMDs. *RMD Open*, *8*(1), Article e002170. https://doi.org/10.1136/rmdopen-2021-002170

Wu, X., Liu, Y., Zou, C., Wang, L., & Zhang, J. (2025). Nicotine's impact on platelet function: Insights into hemostasis mechanisms. *Frontiers in Pharmacology*, *15*, Article 1512142. https://doi.org/10.3389/fphar.2024.1512142

CHAPTER 10

FAQs—Answering Your PRP Questions

Author: Chris Urbanek

What can I expect from PRP?

Earlier in this book, the immediate post-procedure experience was discussed at length, including anticipated soreness, stiffness, the possibility of flares, potential complications, and the initial rest period. The stages of healing and typical patient experiences were also described. But what should you expect beyond this? When can you get back to your goal activity?

Because PRP is a modality that treats the underlying cause and not just the symptoms (like a corticosteroid injection), the onset of relief does take longer as well. If you have had a prior steroid injection, you are likely familiar with the initial relief from the anesthetic. This can take mere minutes and helps to bridge the gap until the steroid starts to work. With PRP treatments, you are typically sorer after the procedure than when you came in. As mentioned earlier, this is an essential part of "calling the workers to the construction site" to start the healing process. Some patients can have a period of notable improvement (to the point of essentially zero pain) immediately after this inflammatory phase. This is not well studied in the literature, but likely represents a period in which the anti-inflammatory cytokines released from the PRP exceed the pro-inflammatory cytokines. While many patients see this as a good thing, it is a period when the patient needs to be extra careful. Do not jump right back into waterskiing when the shoulder feels great 2 weeks after treatment! There simply has not been enough time for actual tissue healing to occur. Full tissue remodeling or healing can take between 8 and 12 weeks, with continued healing that can go beyond this for 6 to even 12 months. Most patients can get back to full activity between 6 and 12 weeks, though there are exceptions, considering the degree of injury, prior baseline level of activity, and the specifics of the goal activity. It is important to discuss with your physician the anticipated outcomes based on your desired goals. While PRP is an effective treatment modality for most conditions, it is not a panacea and cannot fix everything. Setting realistic expectations needs to be a part of your treatment consultation.

Beyond the typical stages of wound healing, we must discuss 2 sub-populations in PRP treatment: the non-responder and the delayed responder. The best published literature on this phenomenon is regarding knee osteoarthritis. While there is a wide variety in the data, the anticipated outcome is that around 20% of patients treated with PRP will not yield an improvement in symptoms. This is typically seen in patients with more advanced disease and those who are treated with lower-quality PRP preparations. One of the criticisms of this literature is that in many of the study designs, the patients were not optimized for treatment. This means not all potential variables may have been evaluated. However, despite all of this, some patients still may not have a meaningful clinical response. The delayed responder group (another 20%) will still achieve their goal outcome, but it can take longer. Sometimes they will not see any improvement until 12 weeks. This can be frustrating to both patient and physician, but trusting in the process and following treatment recommendations could still yield results.

How many injections will I need?

To answer this question, we have to go back to the early days of PRP for musculoskeletal conditions. Initially, the first systems were only able to process a patient's blood at lower volumes and with a lower concentration of platelets. This required more injections to reach some threshold for therapeutic outcome. Now that the technology has improved, it is possible to achieve a therapeutic response with a single injection. More data exists regarding optimal dosing in knee osteoarthritis than in shoulder pathologies, but some generalities exist and are applicable to different scenarios. Osteoarthritis typically responds to higher concentrations, ligament tears or instability to moderate doses, and tendonitis in the low to moderate range. Unfortunately, terms like "high" and "low" are all relative based on the type of system or lab that is processing the blood product. If your physician is using a system that processes to a higher concentration, a single injection may be all that is required. If the concentration is lower, multiple doses may be required. Ultimately, there is no cookie-cutter formula. Every patient responds differently, so treatment needs to be catered to individual responses. Typically, a patient who has good improvement at the 4–6-week mark will have an excellent outcome. If improvement is so-so at 4–6 weeks, you and your physician may consider giving your treatment more time (representing the 20% delayed responder group), or you may opt for a repeat injection. A patient who fails to have any relief by week 8–12 weeks is typically considered to be a non-responder.

What if PRP doesn't work?

As mentioned above, PRP is an individualized treatment approach. Not just in the preparation or injection, but in how the entire patient is treated. Depending on the condition, other treatment options do exist. But these also depend on the patient. What's their candidacy or willingness to pursue other treatments? A patient with severe shoulder osteoarthritis may elect to proceed with a shoulder replacement. However, another patient with the same condition may not be a surgical candidate or may not be willing to proceed with surgery. After a discussion of risks, this may be the most appropriate use for corticosteroid injections–simply to palliate pain. But what if they're an uncontrolled diabetic?! You can see how every aspect of the patient's health has to be considered in directing treatment from the orthobiologic perspective. In a patient who's a good PRP candidate and wants to continue with orthobiologics after a PRP treatment that had some improvement but not to the treatment goal, other cellular injections may be considered, like bone marrow aspirate concentrate (BMAC) or microfragmented adipose (MFAT). These are treatments that utilize another set of your body's cells, different from platelets. Colloquially, these are called stem cells, but there is some argument in the field regarding the accuracy of the term. These injections can be more biologically stimulating and have the potential to yield greater outcomes, though the data is not conclusive. See Table 9.2 summarizing other treatment options. There are certain conditions that are "red flags" necessitating surgical management. These would include full-thickness rotator cuff tears, inflammatory/septic joints, fractures, avascular necrosis, Charcot joints, and dislocations with unstable reduction, to name a few. With multiple options available, it's important to team with your physician to get you the best possible outcome. Treating what are oftentimes complex musculoskeletal conditions is a process that you don't have to navigate alone.

Myths and Misperceptions About PRP

Myth #1: "PRP is just a placebo."

There are multiple peer-reviewed studies demonstrating the effectiveness of PRP for shoulder conditions. The greatest outcomes are with adhesive capsulitis and rotator cuff pathology. While evidence exists for shoulder osteoarthritis, it is not as robust as what exists for other joints, particularly the knee.

Myth #2: "PRP works instantly."

As discussed above, because PRP addresses the underlying tissue pathology and doesn't simply block pain, PRP takes longer to work. Many studies outline the anticipated timeline. To summarize, some patients will note pain relief as early as two weeks, but 8–12 weeks is a typical timeframe for tissue healing.

Myth #3: "PRP is only for athletes."

Absolutely not! PRP can be used in patients of any age. However, as we discussed previously, every treatment needs to be individualized to the patient. The goals of the patient and anticipated outcomes need to be congruent. PRP has to be appropriate for the severity of the condition. Age plays a role as well. There are studies showing that as age increases, PRP outcomes decrease, but it's not just the number! With increasing age comes more wear and tear to the joint or tendon, as well as patients accumulating other medical conditions that may decrease the efficacy of the treatment. This is easily remedied by increasing the concentration of PRP, again on a case-by-case basis.

Top 5 Most Frequently Asked Questions

1. Is PRP safe?

Yes! PRP has a long-standing safety record that exceeds the

safety profile of other injections like corticosteroids.

2. Is PRP effective for partial-thickness rotator cuff tears?

Yes! The data show that PRP can provide statistically significant improvement in both pain and function for both rotator cuff tendonitis and partial-thickness tears. The data is less robust for larger or complete tears.

3. Is PRP better than steroid injections?

Yes! But only if your definition of "better" is in regard to long-term improvement. If you need a "quick fix" to get you through an upcoming vacation or social gathering, steroids have a quicker onset of action and may be more appropriate than PRP depending on timing. Where steroids fail, and PRP dominates, is in long-term outcomes, significantly fewer side effects, and actually healing the underlying tissue.

4. Can I have PRP multiple times before surgery?

Yes! Physiologically, there's no real limit on how many times you can have PRP. Many patients can avoid surgery altogether with repeated treatments when the pain returns. And if you do ultimately have to have surgery, the tissue that the surgeon will be working with is going to be stronger, given the PRP treatment. In fact, some surgeons are utilizing PRP in the operating room at the time of the surgery.

5. Is PRP covered by insurance?

Unfortunately, no. At the time of this writing, no insurance company has PRP listed as a covered treatment. As evidence for superior effectiveness and safety continues to grow, insurance carriers will recognize the benefit of cost savings and harm reduction.

Success Stories and Patient Testimonials

With the vast experience of the writing group behind this text, there are countless success stories that we'd like to share. While there isn't enough space for all of them, a couple are worth highlighting.

One that jumps to mind immediately was a patient of mine who was working in our billing department. Shoulder pain had tortured her for years, and she had been seeing an orthopedic surgeon during this time. Her MRI showed no arthritis, no frozen shoulder, no rotator cuff tear, but there was mild rotator cuff tendonitis. She had been getting multiple steroid injections over the years, "into the bursa," without ultrasound guidance, and pointed to multiple sites around her shoulder. None provided a notable improvement. She had tried PT but was limited by pain. Her goal was to be able to reach into her cabinet so she could bake cookies. On my exam, she had significantly reduced external rotation and a painful and weak rotator cuff exam consistent with her MRI. She clinically had adhesive capsulitis despite a lack of evidence for this on her MRI, but never addressed by her surgeon because it wasn't on the MRI. We established a plan together: ultrasound-guided PRP injection into the shoulder joint to stretch the frozen shoulder, accompanied by a nerve block to stop the pain immediately, followed by physical therapy and a 4-week follow-up to assess her progress and the rotator cuff. At follow-up, she still had pain from the rotator cuff, but not frozen shoulder pain, and her range of motion was significantly improved. A quick PRP injection into the rotator cuff again, with a nerve block to facilitate PT, and after another 4 weeks, her symptoms were resolved. Her multiple-year-long shoulder pain was fixed with a thorough exam and a treatment plan directed at her specific findings.

Another was a patient who presented to the clinic with painful popping when he would throw a ball with his 10-year-old son. It had gotten to the point that he had to stop playing catch in the back yard and avoid any throwing when helping to coach his son's baseball team. He had seen an orthopedic surgeon who tried PT and steroid injections without relief. MRI showed degenerative change of the labrum without a tear. He was told there was nothing more that could be done. His exam was essentially normal *except* that all of his joints were slightly stretcher than they should be. He had an underlying joint hypermobility that was missed by his surgeon. Again, we developed a plan: ultrasound-guided treatment of the inside of the joint where the labrum lives, the labrum itself, AND the ligaments and tendons around the shoulder that provide stability. After treatment, he immediately commented on how stiff and tight the shoulder felt. He had been living with mild instability for years, so a stable joint was a new sensation again. After 6 weeks of physical therapy, the pain and popping were gone, and he was throwing a ball with his son and team again. Why wasn't physical therapy effective initially? His condition was the equivalent of a car having uneven tire wear due to loose struts. You can replace the tires as many times as you want, and they'll still wear unevenly. It's not until you tighten down the struts (restabilize the joint) that the tire wear stops.

Final Takeaway

The response following PRP treatment can be longer than most patients would expect. Prior treatments like NSAIDs and steroid injections perpetuate a false narrative that the onset of relief can be quick. These treatments only block the pain sensations without doing anything to fix the underlying problem. When using PRP to treat an underlying musculoskeletal condition, the pain relief can take several weeks, but the benefit is healthier tissue with longer-lasting improvement and fewer side effects. Persistence with physical therapy, diet, and lifestyle changes, along with patience for the process, is the best formula for success. Utilize your physician as a partner in your care who will follow you through the journey and celebrate your success at the end.

Table 10.1 Shoulder Pathology Treatments

Treatment Option	Mechanism/Explanation	Potential Risks
Physical Therapy	Typically first-line; improves pain, ROM, strength, function; non-invasive	Minimal
NSAIDs	Symptomatic pain relief, anti-inflammatory	Gastrointestinal, Renal, Cardiovascular risks
Corticosteroid Injection	Potent anti-inflammatory; rapid pain relief	Tendon weakening, increased infection risk if surgery within 3 months; systemic effects
Hyaluronic Acid Injection	Viscosupplementation; limited evidence for the shoulder	Local reaction/flare
Surgical Repair (Rotator Cuff)	Tendon reattachment; may use PRP augmentation	Surgical risks; PRP may reduce retear rate but not clinical outcomes
Arthroplasty (Shoulder OA)	Joint replacement for pain and function	Surgical risks
Other Biologics (e.g., BMAC/MFAT)	Cellular therapy utilizing "stem cells."	More invasive, expensive
Neuroablation	Destruction of nerves sending pain signals	Invasive, may require multiple treatments, may also destroy or impair nerves responsible for motion

Bibliography

Baksh, N., Hannon, C. P., Murawski, C. D., Smyth, N. A., & Kennedy, J. G. (2013). Platelet-rich plasma in tendon models: A systematic review of basic science literature. *Arthroscopy: The Journal of Arthroscopic & Related Surgery*, *29*(3), 596–607. https://doi.org/10.1016/j.arthro.2012.10.025

Caplan, A. I. (2010). What's in a name?. *Tissue Engineering Part A*, *16*(8), 2415–2417. https://doi.org/10.1089/ten.TEA.2010.0216

Centeno, C. J., Al-Sayegh, H., Bashir, J., Goodyear, S., & Freeman, M. D. (2015). A prospective multi-site registry study of a specific protocol of autologous bone marrow concentrate for the treatment of shoulder rotator cuff tears and osteoarthritis. *Journal of Pain Research*, *8*, 269–276. https://doi.org/10.2147/JPR.S80872

Chalidis, B., Givissis, P., Papadopoulos, P., & Pitsilos, C. (2023). Molecular and biologic effects of platelet-rich plasma (PRP) in ligament and tendon healing and regeneration: A systematic review. *International Journal of Molecular Sciences*, *24*(3), Article 2744. https://doi.org/10.3390/ijms24032744

Chen, X., Jones, I. A., Togashi, R., Park, C., & Vangsness, C. T., Jr. (2020). Use of platelet-rich plasma for the improvement of pain and function in rotator cuff tears: A systematic review and meta-analysis with bias assessment. *The American Journal of Sports Medicine*, *48*(8), 2028–2041.

https://doi.org/10.1177/0363546519881423

Chowdhary, K., Sahu, A., Iijima, H., Shinde, S., Borg-Stein, J., & Ambrosio, F. (2023). Aging affects the efficacy of platelet-rich plasma treatment for osteoarthritis. *American Journal of Physical Medicine & Rehabilitation*, *102*(7), 597–604. https://doi.org/10.1097/PHM.0000000000002161

Delgado, D., Garate, A., Sánchez, P., Bilbao, A., de Jesus, M. V., & Sánchez, M. (2020). Biological and structural effects after intraosseous infiltrations of age-dependent platelet-rich plasma: An in vivo study. *Journal of Orthopaedic Research*, *38*(9), 1931–1941. https://doi.org/10.1002/jor.24646

Evanson, J. R., Guyton, M. K., Oliver, D. L., Radomski, J. W., & Harrison, A. Z. (2014). Gender and age differences in growth factor concentrations from platelet-rich plasma in adults. *Military Medicine*, *179*(7), 799–805. https://doi.org/10.7205/MILMED-D-13-00336

Hamid, M. S. A., & Sazlina, S. G. (2021). Platelet-rich plasma for rotator cuff tendinopathy: A systematic review and meta-analysis. *PLoS One*, *16*(5), Article e0251111. https://doi.org/10.1371/journal.pone.0251111

Hurley, E. T., Danilkowicz, R. M., & Klifto, C. S. (2023). Editorial commentary: Platelet-rich plasma injections produced a significant improvement in most patients with rotator cuff tendinopathy. *Arthroscopy: The Journal of Arthroscopic & Related Surgery*, *39*(9),

2009–2011. https://doi.org/10.1016/j.arthro.2023.03.022

Lin, H. W., Tam, K. W., Liou, T. H., Rau, C. L., Huang, S. W., & Hsu, T. H. (2023). Efficacy of platelet-rich plasma injection on range of motion, pain, and disability in patients with adhesive capsulitis: A systematic review and meta-analysis. *Archives of Physical Medicine and Rehabilitation*, *104*(12), 2109–2122. https://doi.org/10.1016/j.apmr.2023.03.032

Moraes, V. Y., Lenza, M., Tamaoki, M. J., Faloppa, F., & Belloti, J. C. (2014). Platelet-rich therapies for musculoskeletal soft tissue injuries. *Cochrane Database of Systematic Reviews*, *2014*(4), Article CD010071. https://doi.org/10.1002/14651858.CD010071.pub3

Nudelman, B., Song, B., Higginbotham, D. O., Piple, A. S., & Montgomery, W. H., 3rd. (2023). Platelet-rich plasma injections for shoulder adhesive capsulitis are at least equivalent to corticosteroid or saline solution injections: A systematic review of prospective cohort studies. *Arthroscopy: The Journal of Arthroscopic & Related Surgery*, *39*(5), 1320–1329. https://doi.org/10.1016/j.arthro.2023.01.013

Omid, R., Lalezari, R., Bolia, I. K., & Weber, A. E. (2022). Platelet-rich plasma in the management of shoulder disorders: Basic science and implications beyond the rotator cuff. *Journal of the American Academy of Orthopaedic Surgeons*, *30*(19), e1217–e1226.

https://doi.org/10.5435/JAAOS-D-22-00066

Pang, L., Xu, Y., Li, T., Li, Y., Zhu, J., & Tang, X. (2023). Platelet-rich plasma injection can be a viable alternative to corticosteroid injection for conservative treatment of rotator cuff disease: A meta-analysis of randomized controlled trials. *Arthroscopy: The Journal of Arthroscopic & Related Surgery, 39*(2), 402–421.e1. https://doi.org/10.1016/j.arthro.2022.06.022

Peng, Y., Li, F., Ding, Y., & Chen, J. (2023). Comparison of the effects of platelet-rich plasma and corticosteroid injection in rotator cuff disease treatment: A systematic review and meta-analysis. *Journal of Shoulder and Elbow Surgery, 32*(6), 1303–1313. https://doi.org/10.1016/j.jse.2023.01.037

Prodromos, C. C., Finkle, S., Prodromos, A., Chen, J. L., Schwartz, A., & Wathen, L. (2021). Treatment of rotator cuff tears with platelet rich plasma: A prospective study with 2 year follow-up. *BMC Musculoskeletal Disorders, 22*(1), Article 499. https://doi.org/10.1186/s12891-021-04288-4

Rossi, L. A., Piuzzi, N. S., & Shapiro, S. A. (2020). Glenohumeral osteoarthritis: The role for orthobiologic therapies: Platelet-rich plasma and cell therapies. *JBJS Reviews, 8*(2), Article e0075. https://doi.org/10.2106/JBJS.RVW.19.00075

Tian, J., Lei, X. X., Xuan, L., Tang, J. B., & Cheng, B. (2019). The effects of aging, diabetes mellitus, and antiplatelet drugs on growth factors and anti-aging proteins in platelet-rich plasma. *Platelets, 30*(6), 773–792. https://doi.org/10.1080/09537104.2018.1514110

Tian, J., Li, X. J., Ma, Y., Tang, J. B., Xuan, L., & Cheng, B. (2023). Correlation of bioactive components of platelet rich plasma derived from human female adult peripheral blood and umbilical cord blood with age. *Scientific Reports, 13*(1), Article 18428. https://doi.org/10.1038/s41598-023-45747-3

UW Medicine Family Medicine. (2025). *Regenerative medicine.* UW Medicine Sports Medicine Clinic. https://familymedicine.uw.edu/sports-medicine/patients/regenerative-medicine/

Valencia, R., Anche, G., Cao, V., & Patel, N. (2025). Comparative efficacy of platelet rich plasma, hyaluronic acid, and corticosteroid injections in adhesive capsulitis management: A meta-analysis. *PM&R*. Advance online publication. https://doi.org/10.1002/pmrj.13376

Vaquerizo, V., García-López, M., Mena-Rosón, A., Prado, R., Padilla, S., & Anitua, E. (2023). Plasma rich in growth factors versus corticosteroid injections for management of chronic rotator cuff tendinopathy: A prospective double-blind randomized controlled trial with 1 year of follow-up. *Journal of Shoulder and Elbow Surgery, 32*(3), 555–564. https://doi.org/10.1016/j.jse.2022.08.017

Wang, C., Xu, M., Guo, W., Wang, Y., Zhao, S., & Zhong, L.

(2019). Clinical efficacy and safety of platelet-rich plasma in arthroscopic full-thickness rotator cuff repair: A meta-analysis. *PLoS One*, *14*(7), Article e0220392. https://doi.org/10.1371/journal.pone.0220392

Xiang, X. N., Deng, J., Liu, Y., Yu, X., Cheng, B., & He, H. C. (2021). Conservative treatment of partial-thickness rotator cuff tears and tendinopathy with platelet-rich plasma: A systematic review and meta-analysis. *Clinical Rehabilitation*, *35*(12), 1661–1673. https://doi.org/10.1177/02692155211011944

Zhang, W. B., Ma, Y. L., Lu, FL., Guo, H. R., Song, H., & Hu, Y. M. (2024). The clinical efficacy and safety of platelet-rich plasma on frozen shoulder: A systematic review and meta-analysis of randomized controlled trials. *BMC Musculoskeletal Disorders*, *25*(1), Article 718. https://doi.org/10.1186/s12891-024-07629-1

Zhu, P., Wang, Z., Li, H., & Cai, Y. (2022). Platelet-rich plasma injection in non-operative treatment of partial-thickness rotator cuff tears: A systematic review and meta-analysis. *Journal of Rehabilitation Medicine*, *54*, Article jrm00312. https://doi.org/10.2340/jrm.v54.1434

CHAPTER 11

Managing Shoulder Health Long-Term

Authors: Steve Schaaf & Austin J Sturdivant

Maintaining Shoulder Function after PRP

Platelet-Rich Plasma (PRP) can be a valuable option for many shoulder conditions, especially when paired with a thoughtful rehabilitation plan. Throughout this book, we've discussed PRP's potential to improve pain and function in conditions such as rotator cuff tendinopathy and partial tears, glenohumeral osteoarthritis, subacromial bursitis, adhesive capsulitis (frozen shoulder), labral tears, and even in select cases following shoulder surgery. PRP helps modulate harmful inflammation and jump-start an appropriate healing response in injured soft tissues. While more high-quality research is still needed, current evidence supports PRP's use, particularly for longer-term symptom improvement. As utilization and supportive data continue to grow, so does the importance of a structured rehabilitation after injection.

PRP contains a concentrated mix of growth factors (TGF-B, PDGF, etc.) that promote tissue healing when delivered to the site of injury. PRP can "restart" the healing process, and therapy maintains that progress by applying the right stress at the right time to encourage healthy soft-tissue remodeling. Done appropriately, this combination maximizes shoulder motion and strength long-term.

- Research shows better 1-year pain and function outcomes from a single PRP injection compared with a single corticosteroid injection.
- A meta-analysis of PRP used after shoulder surgery found benefits in most studies, typically alongside standard post-operative rehab that includes stretching and strengthening.
- PRP may be useful for patients who cannot tolerate corticosteroids or who wish to reduce oral pain medication use.
- For partial-thickness rotator cuff tears, PRP can provide clinically meaningful pain relief at medium and long-term (1-year) follow-up. Although the study did point out some limitations in functional gains, reinforcing the need for continued therapy post-injection to optimize function.

Home Exercise and Physical Therapy

A consistent home exercise program (HEP) or physical therapy plan improves function and reduces pain after injection or as a standalone approach. Strengthening at least 2–3 times per week alongside stretching and manual therapy tends to produce the greatest gains in range of motion and function. Tailored programs that combine stretching and strengthening can improve function and quality of life even in irreparable rotator cuff injuries. The same principles apply following PRP injections to further promote healing.

Getting Started

Many patients benefit from a formal physical therapy evaluation before beginning a HEP. Start with a gentle passive range of motion with progression to isometric strengthening. Avoid dynamic movements or heavy lifting that could aggravate symptoms or delay healing. The overarching goal is to stabilize the shoulder while restoring motion, balance strength, and optimize biomechanics.

A Practical Post-PRP Timeline

- **Week 0–1:** Avoid stressful activity to limit excess inflammation. Begin gentle passive ROM, light mobility work, and comfortable upper-extremity cardiovascular exercise.
- **Weeks 1–3:** Progress to active-assisted and then active ROM, restoring mobility without overloading healing tissues. A detailed HEP provides a safe framework.
- **Weeks 2–4:** If pain and function are improving, start light strengthening with isometrics and then advance to isotonic loading as tolerated.
- **Weeks 4–8:** Gradual return to full activity. Sport-specific work depends on the specific injury, mechanism, tissue state, and individual progress. Emphasize range of motion, dynamic stability, and balanced strength. For overhead athletes, follow a graded return-to-throw plan with professional guidance as needed.

Long-Term Maintenance

Because the shoulder is highly mobile and relies on

coordinated muscle support (rotator cuff and scapular stabilizers-trapezius, rhomboids, serratus anterior, levator scapulae), long-term health depends on cross-training (resistance work, pliability/mobility, and cardiovascular training), load management (matching cumulative stress with recovery), and early attention to fatigue or form breakdown to prevent overuse issues.

Preventing Future Shoulder Injuries

Prevention starts with daily mechanics and training habits, especially for people with repetitive shoulder demands.

Ergonomics and Posture

Arrange your work and home environments to support neutral alignment with screens at eye level, supportive seating, and frequently used items within comfortable reach. Targeted neck and shoulder stretching programs have been shown to improve pain and quality of life in office workers. Maintaining neutral posture reduces unnecessary load on scapular stabilizers and the rotator cuff, helping prevent shoulder impingement, muscle imbalance, and altered joint mechanics. Pay attention to sleep position and driving posture as well.

Exercise Form and Warm-Up

For strength training to be beneficial long-term, form matters. Keep the shoulder blades retracted and depressed during upper-body work, avoid excessive elbow flare, and accompany shoulder internal rotation to ensure appropriate joint loading. Evidence suggests Kinesio taping and cold therapy can help with pain and function during rehab for rotator cuff tendinopathy. For overhead shoulder exercises, it is important to maintain a neutral spine, engage the core, and avoid hyperextension of the lower back or letting the arms drift too far behind the head. Always perform a purposeful warm-up with progressive thoracic/shoulder mobility, rotator cuff activation, and scapular stabilization prior to loading the shoulder.

When to Recheck

Seek reevaluation if pain escalates, function (ROM/strength) worsens, or daily/sport tasks become more difficult. New neurologic symptoms (numbness, tingling, weakness) or signs of infection (increased swelling, warmth, redness) warrant prompt medical assessment.

Long-Term Checklist for Shoulder Health

A simple, sustainable plan helps maintain gains and prevent reinjury, especially following a PRP injection.

Strength and Stability (2–3x/week)

- Prioritize high-quality movement and avoid compensatory movements.
- Include resistance-based work (e.g., bands) to build strength and mobility
- Add scapular stabilization exercises to general shoulder programs; this will improve strength, reduce dyskinesis, and help prevent reinjury.

Mobility and Stretching (most days)

- Focus on posture, gentle end-range work, and controlled tempo.
- Goals: maintain ROM, prevent stiffness/contracture, and support circulation to reduce inflammation and pain.

Nutrition, Supplementation, and Hydration (daily)

- Emphasize an anti-inflammatory diet including lean proteins, fruits/vegetables, and omega-3 fats.

- Omega-3s (from foods like salmon, walnuts, or fish-oil supplements) can support cardiometabolic health and lipid profiles.
- There is also evidence to support vitamin C and magnesium, which come along with vitamin D supplementation to support musculoskeletal soft tissue and help prevent injuries.
- Limit processed foods, saturated fats, added sugars, and excess alcohol.
- Stay well hydrated to support joint lubrication, nutrient delivery, and tissue repair.

Annual Check-Up

- Consider yearly follow-ups with a sports medicine physician or physical therapist, especially if you have a history of a shoulder injury, to screen biomechanics and address early warning signs.

Encouragement & Closing Thoughts

Recovery takes time and is rarely linear. From the first weeks after PRP to a return to daily activities or sport, persistence and support make the difference. Your timeline will be unique. Stay connected with your healthcare team, ask questions, and celebrate progress along the way.

Long-term shoulder health is the goal for every patient who has experienced a shoulder injury. Take ownership of your plan: maintain your HEP, stay active, nourish your body, and keep up with periodic check-ins. These habits help you protect your gains and reduce the risk of injury.

For those who have struggled despite conservative care, PRP can offer a path forward. Share your experiences and outcomes with your care team. Your story contributes to the broader understanding of what works best for patients.

Bibliography

Challoumas, D., Biddle, M., McLean, M., & Millar, N. L. (2020). Comparison of treatments for frozen shoulder: A systematic review and meta-analysis. *JAMA Network Open, 3*(12), Article e2029581. https://doi.org/10.1001/jamanetworkopen.2020.29581

Christensen, B. H., Andersen, K. S., Rasmussen, S., Andreasen, L. L., Nielsen, L. M., & Jensen, S. L. (2016). Enhanced function and quality of life following 5 months of exercise therapy for patients with irreparable rotator cuff tears - an intervention study. *BMC Musculoskeletal Disorders, 17*, Article 252. https://doi.org/10.1186/s12891-016-1116-6

Desouza, C., & Shetty, V. (2024). Effectiveness of platelet-rich plasma in partial-thickness rotator cuff tears: A systematic review. *Journal of ISAKOS, 9*(4), 699–708. https://doi.org/10.1016/j.jisako.2024.04.010

Durgut, E., Gurses, H. N., Bilsel, K., Alpay, K., Hosbay, Z., Uzer, G., Yıldız, F., & Elmalı, N. (2024). Short-term effects of cold therapy and Kinesio taping on pain relief and upper extremity functionality in individuals with rotator cuff tendonitis: A randomized study. *Medicina, 60*(8), Article 1188. https://doi.org/10.3390/medicina60081188

Kuszewski, J. C., Wong, R. H. X., Wood, L. G., & Howe, P. R. C. (2020). Effects of fish oil and curcumin supplementation on cerebrovascular function in older adults: A randomized controlled trial. *Nutrition, Metabolism and Cardiovascular Diseases, 30*(4), 625–633. https://doi.org/10.1016/j.numecd.2019.12.010

Rossi, L. A., Brandariz, R., Gorodischer, T., Camino, P., Piuzzi, N., Tanoira, I., & Ranalletta, M. (2024). Subacromial injection of platelet-rich plasma provides greater improvement in pain and functional outcomes compared to corticosteroids at 1-year follow-up: A double-blinded randomized controlled trial. *Journal of Shoulder and Elbow Surgery, 33*(12), 2563–2571. https://doi.org/10.1016/j.jse.2024.06.012

Shen, Z., Ye, X., He, Y., Shen, G., Xu, K., Zhang, B., & Wu, L. (2024). Arthroscopic rotator cuff repair combined with platelet-rich plasma products can reduce the rate of retearing and improve clinical outcomes: A meta-analysis of randomized controlled trials. *Medicine, 103*(18), Article e38069. https://doi.org/10.1097/MD.0000000000038069

Thu, A. C., Kwak, S. G., Shein, W. N., Htun, M., Htwe, T. T. H., & Chang, M. C. (2020). Comparison of ultrasound-guided platelet-rich plasma injection and conventional physical therapy for management of adhesive capsulitis: A randomized trial. *Journal of International Medical Research, 48*(12), Article 300060520976032. https://doi.org/10.1177/0300060520976032

Tunwattanapong, P., Kongkasuwan, R., & Kuptniratsaikul, V.

(2016). The effectiveness of a neck and shoulder stretching exercise program among office workers with neck pain: A randomized controlled trial. *Clinical Rehabilitation*, *30*(1), 64–72. https://doi.org/10.1177/0269215515575747

Yuksel, E., & Yesilyaprak, S. S. (2024). Scapular stabilization exercise training improves treatment effectiveness on shoulder pain, scapular dyskinesis, muscle strength, and function in patients with subacromial pain syndrome: A randomized controlled trial. *Journal of Bodywork and Movement Therapies*, *37*, 101–108. https://doi.org/10.1016/j.jbmt.2023.11.005

CONCLUSION

Shoulder pain can have a profound impact on daily life, affecting work, recreation, sleep, and overall quality of life. Fortunately, advances in musculoskeletal medicine have expanded the range of treatment options available to patients. Platelet-rich plasma (PRP) has emerged as one such option, offering a biologic approach that utilizes components derived from a patient's own blood. As research continues to evolve, PRP has demonstrated promising results for select shoulder conditions, including tendinopathies, partial-thickness rotator cuff tears, adhesive capsulitis, and osteoarthritis.

Throughout this book, we have explored the anatomy of the shoulder, common causes of shoulder pain, the science behind PRP, current clinical evidence, treatment expectations, and rehabilitation principles. While PRP is not a cure-all and may not be appropriate for every patient or diagnosis, it represents an important addition to the continuum of care between conservative treatment measures and surgery. Appropriate patient selection, accurate diagnosis, image-guided injection techniques, and adherence to rehabilitation protocols remain critical factors in achieving the best possible outcomes.

Healthcare decisions are most effective when patients are informed and actively involved in their care. We hope this book has provided you with a better understanding of PRP and its potential role in managing shoulder pain. Whether you ultimately choose physical therapy, medications, injections, surgery, PRP, or a combination of treatments, our goal is that you feel empowered to have informed discussions with your healthcare team and make decisions that align with your individual needs, goals, and lifestyle.

The field of orthobiologics continues to advance rapidly, and future research will further refine our understanding of how biologic therapies can be used to help patients maintain function and improve quality of life. Until then, a thoughtful, evidence-based approach remains the foundation of high-quality patient care.

Thank you for allowing us to be part of your educational journey. We wish you success in your pursuit of improved shoulder health, function, and return to the activities that matter most to you.

www.ingramcontent.com/pod-product-compliance
Lightning Source LLC
LaVergne TN
LVHW020233210926
848481LV00015B/1780
9798996347513